I0492286

DIABETES AND OTHER CHRONIC DISEASES
ЯEVERSED:
The drug-free remedy.

Published By:

Dr. J. L. Mulatya

ISBN 979-8685-184-82-5

First Published 2020

Preface

In 1903, DR Thomas A Addison said "The doctor of the future will give no medication, but will interest his patients in the care of the human frame, diet, and in the cause and prevention of disease".

More than a century later, the opposite is happening. There is a global decline in morbidity and mortality due to Communicable Diseases, and an increase in the burden of Non-Communicable Diseases (NCDs). We are facing the biggest epidemic of preventable NCDs in human history.

In 2020, World Health Organization (WHO) estimates that 2/3 of all diseases will be lifestyle diseases. The global epidemic of Obesity, Diabetes Mellitus, Cardiovascular Disease, hypertension, cancer etc. is related to dietary guidelines.

The fact that diabetes Type-2 is reversible is no longer debatable. Some cancers and refractory epilepsy respond to diet better than any other known treatment modality.

This book takes you through my personal journey to Diabetes Type-2 Reversal, the results of a low-carbohydrate high-fat diet (LCHF) Observational Study, the myths, the various clinical applications, challenges in implementation, Anesthetic considerations, medico-legal aspects, economic impacts and future of the LCHF diets.

This Book is for the following:

1. The ordinary patient with a chronic disease e.g. Diabetes, Hypertension, Obesity, Alzheimer's disease, Arthritis etc. who wants to know the other Option.

2. The Nutritionist/Dietician disappointed by Disease outcomes.

3. The Physician who believes in the mantra; Let food be thy Medicine.

4. The Gynecologist who wants the safest/effective treatment for PCOS.

5. The Pediatrician/Neurologist with that Refractory Epileptic Child/Adult.

6. The Pregnant/Lactating mother who wants to know what to eat.

7. The Oncologist/Cancer patient who wants Sole treatment/ adjuvant to Chemotherapy and or Radiotherapy.

8. The Non-Communicable Disease Policy Makers.

9. The Medical Insurer who wants to reduce Medical Claims.

10. The Anesthetist who wants safety during Anesthesia.

11. The Medical doctor/Academician who wants to broaden his knowledge on this topic which is hardly covered in Undergraduate and Postgraduate Curriculum.

12. The Athlete who wants to increase his physical endurance.

13. Anybody who wants to achieve good health and longevity.

Acknowledgements:

I acknowledge the immense contribution of:

1. My wife Lucy Wanza Mulatya for her support during my journey to Diabetes Type-2 reversal, during the Observational Study and in the Typing of the manuscript.

2. Many colleagues globally who have contributed in scientific journals, books and conferences on LCHF diets.

3. The patients whose response to the LCHF diets has been very encouraging.

4. All Staff of MULATYA MEMORIAL HOSPITAL, MAKUENI COUNTY, KENYA.

5. South African Professor Tim Noakes and the NUTRITION NETWORK TEAM for their Online Learning Platform.

6. My Sister Jacinta Mulatya for her prayers and typing of the Manuscript.

BE BLESSED!

Published by:
Dr. Mulatya
Mulatya Memorial Hospital
P.O. Box 75 - 90138,
Makindu, Kenya.

jlmulatya@gmail.com

Typesetting and lay-out: **Bryan Mwaniki** *(Refined Concepts)*

TABLE OF CONTENTS

FOREWORD
IT TAKES GREAT COURAGE TO CHANGE

It takes great courage to change one's mind. Not least to question a conviction that one has trusted and religiously followed for all of one's professional career. And on which one has based the management of patients who have placed their faith in you, the doctor, in the belief that you will always practice, and deliver, what is in *their* best interests.

But there may well come that moment when that doctor is forced to face an uncomfortable truth. When the trusted expert becomes aware, painfully at first, that some of what he or she professes, is not just plainly wrong. But also, harmful. That the trust the patients have placed in their healer, is misplaced. And it is then that the great doctors, the very best, instinctively know that whatever the cost to their pride and ego, they must acknowledge their error. They must reject much of what they formerly believed and, instead, embrace a novel truth.

Dr J.L. Mulatya is one of those great doctors who, when faced with that moment of truth, did not falter. Instead, he swallowed his pride and chose the path of humility and righteousness.

Dr Mulatya relates that he was born into a well-to-do Kenyan family, the son of a Colonial Chief. He grew up eating the healthy and nutritious Kenyan diet of cooked beans, maize, ugali, and traditional green vegetables, supplemented with occasional beef, goat, mutton, and cows' milk. During the Festive Season, boiled eggs, chicken stew and chapatti were added delicacies.

Large herds of cattle grazed on the lush grasslands and food was plentiful. Diseases were uncommon with the exception of transient fevers as well as measles, whooping cough, and polio, before vaccination became more widespread. Supportive medical care was provided by shrewd traditional healers, whose abilities are generally unappreciated by the paternalistic attitude of conventional Western medicine.

But Dr. Mulatya tells how all that has changed in just one generation. The traditional healthy Kenyan diet of locally-grown foods has been replaced by the foods of the colonists; what Dr. Weston Price called the "displacing foods of modern commerce" (1). With devastating consequences. And Dr. Mulatya himself has been one of its casualties.

So it was that in in 2007 at age 52 years, Dr. Mulatya was faced with the reality that he had developed type 2 diabetes mellitus; a disease which his training would have taught him is progressive, irreversible and leads to an early death from any of a number of different, devastating complications - Like blindness, kidney failure, heart disease, stroke and lower limb gangrene requiring amputation.

For the first year after his diagnosis, Dr. Mulatya followed the standard medical advice. He religiously took his prescribed medications even though they caused him significant side-effects. He followed a low-fat "heart-healthy" diet with limited meat and eggs and in which sugar and sugary drinks were forbidden. But there was no restriction on sweet and sugary fruits; or on carbohydrate-rich vegetables, millet, sorghum, ugali, beans, or peas.

But after his mother died of the complications of type 2 diabetes, Dr. Mulatya was jolted out of his complacency. He realized that if he was to avoid the same fate, he would need to learn more about his disease. He appreciated, dimly at first, that the most effective way for the doctor to learn about any disease is for the doctor to first develop that disease, and to learn how to live with it. But it would take time for the critically important lessons of this particular disease to be learned.

By 2012, five years after his diabetes diagnosis, Dr. Mulatya had developed the first tell-tale signs of poorly controlled diabetes – numbness in his lower limbs indicating the development of diabetic peripheral neuropathy. But the only cure he could find online involved a variety of herbal remedies, none of which worked.

The initial breakthrough came in 2015 when he encountered the TEDx talk by Dr. Sarah Hallberg entitled: *Reversing Type 2 Diabetes Starts by Ignoring The Guidelines*. That presentation attests to the miracle of social media. Already it has been viewed by more than 3 million people. It was the turning point. It opened the doctor's eyes to a world of medicine that he did not know even exists.

But still, he was not yet ready to commit fully to Dr. Hallberg's challenge.

So a year later despite using even more medications, his blood glucose control had become yet more erratic. Although he was following the "healthy" lifestyle including eating the diet prescribed by a Nutritionist according to the Kenya Diabetes Association's Nutrition guidelines; he was exercising regularly and avoiding sugar and alcohol. Yet he continued to carry excess weight.

His moment of truth came in November 2017 when he discovered the Banting low-carbohydrate high-fat diet. Combined with intermittent fasting, he finally began this new method of eating, fully a decade after he had first been diagnosed as a type 2 diabetic.

At first, it was not easy as he had to cope with an overpowering craving for carbohydrates manifested as a range of bodily symptoms. But the positive outcome was that, within days, his severely elevated blood glucose concentrations had fallen dramatically to within the low-normal range. He began removing first one, then two, and ultimately all three of his diabetes medications. Within six weeks, his weight was also within the normal range. As he writes: "the feet numbness…was decreasing, my mood and sleep patterns had greatly improved, the brain frog disappeared; I was strong and energetic the way I used to feel twenty years prior. My vision improved, in less than four months my HbA1c dropped from 9.8 to 5.5%. YES, I HAD REVERSED DIABETES!".

In short Dr. Mulatya had experienced a miracle. A miracle that his profession cannot acknowledge because it conflicts so absolutely with the current medical model of type 2 diabetes as an incurable, progressively fatal condition. The medical profession which, in its ignorance and willful blindness (3) prefers rather to promote an incorrect therapeutic model, using pharmaceutical drugs to "treat" a condition that, as Dr. Mulatya experience shows, is a behavioral disease caused purely by inappropriate food choices.

This book is so important because it uses Dr. Mulatya's personal but anecdotal experiences to introduce the hard science that explains why his personal miracle is not really a miracle at all. It is a miracle only to those who refuse to engage with that hard-won evidence. It is certainly not a miracle to those who understand that it is predicted by the wealth of the science that he has carefully presented in the pages of this book. Dr. Mulatya shows concisely that, thanks to the scientific work of Dr. Hallberg and her colleagues (2) and many others, we now know that type 2 diabetes is eminently "reversible" in the vast majority of sufferers. But only if they understand that the choice is theirs. Eat properly and reverse the disease. It really is that simple.

There is a reason why Dr. Mulatya has been chosen to traverse this difficult and treacherous path. Because what he learned and the message he wishes to present, is so very, very important for the continent of Africa.

The peoples of our continent have struggled for centuries with the ravages of infectious diseases. Now increasingly we are suffering under the added burden of what are incorrectly labelled "chronic diseases of lifestyle". Like obesity, high blood pressure, metabolic syndrome, and diabetes.

But these are *NOT* diseases of lifestyle; they *ARE* diseases of nutrition as Dr. Mulatya's experience clearly shows. And if all are diseases of *nutrition* then their prevention and cure must be a *nutritional* one – exactly as Dr. Mulatya's experience proves to be the case.

But the only way that we can ever promote a nutritional solution for these nutritional diseases is if we radically alter the way medicine is taught on our continent. We need to return to the eating patterns we once followed when these nutritional diseases had not yet been encountered by African peoples.

This book promises a new start.

It must be in every medical school library across the continent; it needs to be in every high school library from Cape to Cairo; from the shores of the Atlantic Ocean in the West to the Indian Ocean in the East.

Dr. Mulatya's courage is his gift to us.

We must not waste it.

Emeritus Professor Timothy Noakes
OMS, MBChB, MD, DSc, PhD (hc), FACSM, (hc) FFSEM UK, (hc) FFSEM (Ire)

References:
1. Price W. *Nutrition and Physical Degeneration: A comparison of Primitive and Modern Diets and Their Effects.* Benediction Classics, United Kingdom. 2010.

2. Hallberg SJ, McKenzie AL, Williams PT, et al. Effectiveness and safety of a novel care model for the management of type 2 diabetes at 1 year: An open-label, non-randomized, controlled study. *Diab Ther* 2018;9:583–612.

3. Heffernan M. *Wilful Blindness. Why we ignore the obvious at our peril.* Ebooksweb. Bensalem PA, USA. 2009

ENDORSEMENTS & READERS' REVIEWS

I congratulate Dr. Mulatya on the extensive work he has done on the role of Low Carbohydrate High Fat (LCHF) diet on non-communicable diseases that have become major causes of morbidity and mortality in our time.

Basing his discourse on positive outcomes of real cases he has handled and on previous findings by many researchers globally, Dr. Mulatya has consolidated the knowledge on LCHF diet providing a rich resource to all who are passionate about dietary interventions. I applaud Dr. Mulatya for being his own testament and a success story whose application of rigorous dietary and lifestyle modifications reversed diabetes.

I recommend this book as an invaluable reference manual and believe it will contribute to greater appreciation for the role of LCHF as well as provoke further research.

Dorothy Mugane,
Public Health & Nutrition Specialist

I have read the book twice. The first time, I went through it to get an understanding of the author's thoughts and the approach, which was different. The second time, I got to understand the full picture and the approach to the author's writing, which is based on a topic (Case presentation) and then followed by an Evidence-Based Medicine (EBM) discussion.

I loved the flow of thoughts since it gives an insight on all the cases and the current thinking in terms of management (LCHF, Keto, etc).

I must say this is a well written book, with all the current Evidence Based Medicine. Excellent work doc!

Dr. Daniel Katambo.
Physician

Book Review: By the Kenya Nutritionists and Dieticians Institute

Low-Carb-Ketogenic Diets(KDs) are characterized by intake of high fat, adequate proteins and very low amounts of carbohydrates. The Carbohydrate intake is usually less than 50g/day. The knowledge regarding the metabolic effects of classic ketogenic diets originates from the pioneering work of Cahill and colleagues in the 1960s but the realization of the importance of these diets from a clinical point of view can be traced back to the early1920s when they began to be successfully used in the treatment of epilepsy. In the recent past, the therapeutic use of ketogenic diets in other diseases has been studied with positive results and is an important direction for research.

There is no doubt that a strong supportive evidence exists on the effectiveness of low carbohydrates ketogenic diet in weight-loss therapy. However, there are contrasting theories regarding the mechanisms through which it works. Some studies suggest that low carbohydrate diets may not have any advantage and that weight loss occurs due to reduction in calorie intake, probably due to the increased satiety effect of protein. A simpler, perhaps more likely, explanation for improved weight loss is a possible appetite-suppressant action of ketosis. The mechanism for this is not established but evidence supports direct action of ketone bodies together with modifications in levels of hormones, which influence appetite, such as ghrelin and leptin.

A number of studies point to beneficial effects of diets low in carbohydrates on cardiovascular risk factors. Although doubts have been expressed on the safety, effectiveness and long-term use of ketogenic diets compared to balanced diets and clearly negative opinions regarding possible deleterious effects on triglycerides and cholesterol levels in the blood. However, a number of recent studies demonstrate that the reduction of carbohydrates to levels that induce physiological ketosis can actually lead to significant benefits in blood lipid profiles The effect of KDs seems to be particularly marked on the level of blood triglycerides but there are also significant positive effects reduction of total cholesterol reduction and increase in high-density lipo protein. Furthermore, KDs have been reported to increase the size and volume of low-density lipoprotein cholesterol particles which is considered to reduce cardiovascular

Insulin resistance is the primary feature underlying type 2 diabetes (T2D) and a person with it will divert a greater proportion of dietary carbohydrate to the liver where much of it is converted to fat through denovolipogenes is as opposed to being oxidized for energy in skeletal muscle. Denovolipogenes is contributes about 20%of new triglycerides, this greater conversion of dietary carbohydrate into fat where much of it enters the circulatory system as saturated fat, is a metabolic abnormality that significantly increases risk for diabetes and heart disease. Therefore, insulin resistance functionally manifests itself as 'carbohydrate intolerance'. Signs and symptoms of insulin resistance improve or disappear when dietary carbohydrate is restricted to a level below which is not significantly converted to fat (a threshold that varies from person to person), signs and symptoms of insulin resistance improve or often disappear completely.

In a longer study, obese T2D individuals were prescribed a well-formulated ketogenic diet for 56weeks, and significant improvements in both weight loss and metabolic parameters were seen at 12 weeks and continued through out the 56 weeks as evidenced by improvements in fasting circulating levels of glucose (51%), total cholesterol (29%), high-density lipoprotein-cholesterol (63%), low-density lipoprotein-cholesterol (33%) and triglycerides (41%).

Although significant reductions in fat mass often results when individuals restrict carbohydrate, the improvements in glycemic control, hemoglobin A1c and lipid markers, as well as reduced use or withdrawal of insulin and other medications in many cases, occurs before significant weight loss occurs. Moreover, in isocaloric experiments individuals with insulin resistance showed dramatically improved markers of metabolic syndrome than diets lower in fat. It is interesting in this respect that a recent extremely large epidemiological study reported that diabetes risk is directly correlated, in an apparently causative manner, with sugar in take alone, independently of weight or sedentary lifestyle. In summary, individuals with metabolic syndrome, insulin resistance and T2D (all diseases of carbohydrate intolerance) are likely to see both symptomatic and objective improvements in bio-markers of disease risk if they follow a well-formulated very low-carbohydrate diet. Glucose control improves not only because there is less glucose coming in, but also because systemic insulin sensitivity improves as well.

Since 1920, the ketogenic diet has been recognized as an effective tool in the treatment of severe childhood epilepsy, but following the introduction of anti-convulsant drugs, the interest in ketogenic diet treatment waned until the1990s, with subsequent research and clinical trials demonstrating its practical usefulness. Various studies have been carried out to understand its mechanism of action in epilepsy, but until now it remains largely uncertain. The effectiveness of ketogenic diets is strongly supported in a recent Cochrane review where all studies showed a 30-40% reduction in seizures compared with comparative controls, and there view authors reported that in children the effects were 'comparable to modern anti-epileptic drugs'. The main draw back with the ketogenic diet is the difficult tolerability and high dropout rates given the extremely positive results and the severe side effects common with anti-epilepsy medication, the development of an easier-to-follow ketogenic diet would be a worthwhile goal. Finally, in as much as Ketogenic diets are commonly considered to be useful remedy for weight control and many studies suggest that they could be more efficient than low-fat diets, there is no concordance in the literature about their absolute effectiveness and even some doubts are raised about safety. But there is a 'hidden face' of the ketogenic diet: its broader therapeutic action. On this matter studies are warranted to investigate more in detail the potential therapeutic mechanisms, its effectiveness and safety. This does not rule out the overall effectiveness on diabetic management in the long run. The issue of sustainability is still a big question to answer in the field of research.

This book therefore highlights some of the benefits of Low-Carbohydrates diet that would give a useful intervention in Diabetes management not forgetting related diseases.

Dr. David Omondi Okeyo,

Msc., PhD, MPH Public Health Nutrition Scientist
Kenya Nutritionists and Dieticians Institute
Affiliate of Maseno University, Kenya

References:

Basu S, Yoffe P, Hills N, Lustig R H. The relationship of sugar to population-level diabetes prevalence: An econometric analysis of repeated cross- sectional data. Plo S One 2013; 8: e57873

Dashti H M, Al-Zaid N S, Mathew T C, Al-Mousawi M, Talib H, Asfar S Ketal. Long term effects of ketogenic diet in obese subjects with high cholesterol level. Mol Cell Biochem 2006; 286:1–9.

Kessler S K, Neal E G, Camfield C S, Kossoff E H. Dietary therapies for epilepsy: future research. Epilepsy Behav 2011;22:17–22

Nielsen J V, Joensson E A. Low-carbohydrate diet in type 2 diabetes:Stable improvement of body weight and glycemic control during 44 months follow-up. Nutr Metab (Lond) 2008;5:14

Jornayvaz F R, Samuel V T, Shulman G I. The role of muscle insulin resistance in the pathogenesis of atherogenic dyslipidemia and non alcoholic fatty liver disease associated with the metabolic syndrome. Annu Rev Nutr 2010; 30:273–290.

Sharman M J, Kraemer W J, Love D M, Avery N G, Gomez A L, Scheett T P etal. A ketogenic diet favorably affects serumbio markers for cardio vascular disease in normal-weight men. J Nutr 2002;132:1879–1885.

Volek J S, Sharman M J, Forsy the CE. Modification of lipoproteins by very low-carbohydrate diets. J Nutr 2005;135:1339–1342

Paoli A, Cenci L, Fancelli M, Parmagnani A, FratterA, Cucchi A etal. Ketogenic diet and phyto extracts comparison of the efficacy of mediterranean, zone and tisanoreica diet on some health risk factors. Agro Food Ind Hi-Tech 010; 21:24

Brehm B J, Seeley R J, Daniels S R, D'Alessio D A. A randomized trial comparing a very low carbohydrate diet and a calorie-restricted low-fatdieton body weight and cardiovascular risk factors in healthy women. J Clin Endocrinol Metab 2003; 88:1617–1623

Blackburn G L, Phillips J C, Morreale S. Physician's guide to popular lowcarbohydrateweight-lossdiets.CleveClinJMed2001;68:761– 766768–9, 773–4

Kessler S K, Neal E G, Camfield C S, Kossoff E H. Dietarytherapiesforepilepsy: future research. Epilepsy Behav 2011; 22:17–22.

Owen O E, Morgan A P, Kemp H G, Sullivan J M, Herrera M G, Cahill Jr G F. Brain metabolism during fasting. J Clin Invest 1967; 46:1589–1595.

Veech R L. The therapeutic implications of ketone bodies: The effects of ketone bodies in pathological conditions: ketosis, ketogenic diet, redoxstates, insulin resistance, and mitochondrial metabolism. Prostaglandins Leukot Essent Fatty Acids 2004; 70:309–319

Nordmann A J, Nordmann A, Briel M, Keller U, Yancy Jr W S, Brehm B J etal. Effects of low-carbohydrate vs low-fat diets on weight loss and cardiovascular risk factors: ameta-analysis of randomized controlled trials. Arch Intern Med 2006; 166:285–293.

Westerterp - Plantenga M S, Nieuwenhuizen A, Tome D, Soenen S, Westerterp KR. Dietary protein, weight loss, and weight maintenance. Annu Rev Nutr 2009; 29:21–41

ShaiI, Schwarzfuchs D, Henkin Y, Shahar D R, Witkow S, Greenberg I etal. Weight loss with a low-carbohydrate, mediterranean, or low-fat diet. N Eng l J Med 2008; 359: 229–241.

Sumithran P, Prendergast L A, Delbridge E, Purcell K, Shulkes A, Kriketos A etal. Ketosis and appetite-mediating nutrients and hormones after weight loss. Eur J Clin Nutr 2013; e-pub ahead of print 1 May 2013; doi:10.1038/ejcn. 2013. 90

INTRODUCTION

The year is 2007. I am a busy Consultant Anesthesiologist working in a government hospital. I notice that I am drinking a lot of water and frequently urinating. For some years I have had frequent skin rashes on the feet and white ulcerations between the toes. Though I use spectacles, my sight is progressively getting worse. I am losing weight and feeling weak. I am 52-year male, slightly obese, stopped drinking alcohol some twenty years ago. I stopped cigarette smoking 7 years ago. Sometimes I work for many hours anaesthetizing patients in the Operating theatres, reviewing Preoperative, Postoperative and Intensive Care Unit (ICU) patients. I am never guaranteed of regular sleep and rarely take part in social activities.

I am married with children, some in universities. My wife understands that we need money to meet family needs including building a family home in a leafy posh suburb.

I was born to a relatively well up Kenyan African family. My father was a Colonial Chief, my mum a career housewife. Although we were a total of eight siblings in the family, we could afford to live in a corrugated iron sheet (*Mabati*) house with a cement floor in a village set up. I attended the local primary school, moved to secondary schools in Kenyan major towns and finally to National University for Medical School Undergraduate studies, and later Postgraduate degree in Anesthesiology.

In the village, our main food was cooked beans and maize '*githeri*', white maize flour 'ugali', traditional green vegetables, occasional beef, goat, mutton, and fresh or fermented cow milk. During the festive season e.g. Christmas, boiled eggs, chicken stew and chapatti was a delicacy to share with visitors.

Life was communal. We knew all our relatives and neighbors. There was plenty of food, diseases were rare; mainly fever – commonly termed as '*ndetema*' which meant every cause of fever and general malaise including malaria. Coughs, constipation, diarrhea and leg ulcers were common. A visit to the local dispensary for the painful Chloroquine injection; a bitter dose of castor oil

'Kasitowelo' for constipation, sulfadiazine *'suta'* capsule, or a visit to the local herbalist for that special herbal root for abdominal pain relief, was all you needed. Wounds would be treated traditionally and successfully with a special sap from local plants such as *'mutungate'* or *'kavete'*.

Children diseases such as measles, whooping cough, and Polio were common. Later, vaccines for these viral infections including smallpox were introduced. Family planning was unknown and mothers would deliver many children to allow for natural selection.

There were no Antenatal clinics. Antenatal care and deliveries were conducted by traditional birth attendants. After delivery, mothers were fed on soup from fattened sheep *'nduume'* and porridge from maize, millet, or sorghum.

Our herbalists used traditional treatments for various diseases; for example, acupuncture or a form of shiatsu therapy *'kukilya kavoo'* for dyspepsia, special herbal leaves, steam inhalation for whooping cough and measles, boiled herbs for arthritis *'mutambuko'* and various herbal treatments for snakebites. In cases of vomiting of blood *'kiathi'*, traditional remedies were available.

A specially-made non-polarizing muscle relaxant (curare) from boiled leaves of a secret plant *'ivai'* was used for hunting big game when applied to arrows.

Modern non-communicable diseases were rare or non-existent. The likes of Diabetes, Hypertension, Obesity, Cancers, Mental illness, Epilepsy, were mostly unheard of. The elderly mostly died of old age and were buried by the younger generation.

According to a Zimbabwean Colonial Medical Practitioner Michael Gelfand in his 1948 book ***"The sick African" (1)***, Africans were portrayed as sick unhealthy people. *He was noted for a humanistic approach to medicine and for his historical and ethnographic works which are considered to have played an important role in his re-examination of significant prejudices he held about African people's culture and religious practices."* Initially, Gelfand held decidedly negative views of African patients and indigenous healers. Later, he began to overcome his earlier prejudices and came to acknowledge that African

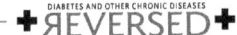
traditional healers were shrewd Herbalists and Psychologists. In 1978, he admitted having initially "accepted the prevailing preconceived idea that all African People were backward and that their religion and much more their code of conduct were primitive, but that through his research he had found that the traditional beliefs of these people were as rational as those of other faiths of the Western World. He eventually discovered that the African diet was balanced, nutritious and not abundant in refined sugars and cholesterol as is the Western diet. The African diet was rich in fiber, and those living on it rarely suffered from peptic ulcers, acute appendicitis, gallstones or even cancer of the large bowel."

Rains were reliable and so were the farm yields in cassava, sorghum, millet, peas, and beans. Land for grazing was available and large herds of cattle were a common sight.

Owning a bicycle was for the privileged few like the much-respected local Primary School Headteacher. Nursery schools were non-existent. English was taught from Standard three, lower Primary classes ended at 11 am and children had time to play, set bird traps, and listen to stories and Folk songs from their grandparents in the evening.

The Agricultural Extension Officer 'ndilikasa' made sure that furrows to prevent soil erosion were made.

Unfortunately, our ways of life have changed. In one generation, we have embraced the modern way of life. Our grazing lands have decreased; the numbers of livestock, farm size, and agricultural productivity have decreased. Traditional crops like cassava, sweet potatoes, and fermented porridge have been forgotten.

Modern eating habits were introduced and embraced. Bread, chapati, rice, processed foods and drinks, kales (sukumawiki), spinach and fast foods have become staples. We lead a sedentary lifestyle compounded by environmental pollutants, stressful conditions, nutritional deficiencies, climate change, medical knowledge geared towards disease treatment rather than prevention, leading to the proliferation of modern-day Non-Communicable diseases (NCDs). It is no wonder that in 2007, I became an additional statistic of Diabetes Mellitus Type-2 (DMT2) in Kenya.

CHAPTER ONE

DIAGNOSIS OF DIABETES

I suspected that I had diabetes due to the rapidly progressing symptoms, excessive thirst and frequent urination. I had developed a craving for sweet foods, especially ice cream and a love for bread with avocado and a lot of honey. I analyzed my genetic predisposition to Diabetes; my mother was diabetic, but I was still in denial. I booked an appointment with a female colleague: An Endocrinologist. A visit to her clinic, short history and examination, a random blood sugar reading of 17 mmol per litre confirmed a diagnosis of Diabetes mellitus. My blood pressure was normal. A battery of Laboratory investigations was ordered; urinalysis, full haemogram, urea and electrolytes, and lipid profile. The results were normal except for glycosuria and high total cholesterol. I was put on oral hypoglycemic agents (OHA); Metformin, Glibenclamide, Pioglitazone and a cholesterol-lowering agent, Atorvastatin. I was booked for a nutrition session later, accompanied by my wife.

As I left the clinic, the world outside had suddenly changed; I was fully in distress. How can I be a diabetic? How is it that I, (a doctor) had ignored all the symptoms of Diabetes, some for years? After all the diabetes complications I had witnessed as a doctor? Patients coming in coma due to low/high blood sugars, hypertension, kidney failure, leg amputations; the list was endless. I wondered; what will I be eating? Will I be able to work and support my family? I realized that a sick medical person suffers more than a non-medical patient when he/she is diagnosed with an illness. You are assumed to know and understand everything concerning the disease and therefore do not require counseling. I felt like half of me had been cut off. I informed my wife about the doctor's findings and started taking the medications as prescribed while waiting for the Nutritionist's appointment. I realized that the medications had side effects; headaches, diarrhea, etc., but at the back of my mind, I knew that diabetes is a chronic progressive disease, and this was the beginning of taking medications throughout my life. I started losing interest in my work, my thought process was slow and disorganized; I was depressed.

Finally, my wife and I had a session with the Nutritionist. I got the conventional diabetes nutritional advice. I was told to: reduce fat intake, eat whole foods (brown rice, bread and brown flat bread 'chapati'), take small quantities of meat, avoid fat, eat preferably skinless chicken, one egg per week, fistful of millet, sorghum or maize flour 'ugali'. For legumes: have beans, peas a serving per meal, adequate fruits and green vegetables, sugarless tea and yogurt. I was advised to avoid sugary drinks and take diet coke if necessary. This sounded easy and straightforward but I realized that the family's meals had to change. If I didn't have good family support, I would have felt both segregated and stigmatized. It was not better at the workplace either, so I had to pack home meals and have them in an isolated place with questions from curious colleagues unanswered.

Between the medications and diet, I felt better and the side effects of the medications reduced gradually. My vision improved and I started gaining weight, the thirst and frequent urination decreased. I slowly accepted my condition and my mood and sleep pattern improved. Clinic follow-up and laboratory results confirmed that my DMT2 was well-controlled. Less than a year after I was confirmed to be diabetic my mother succumbed to diabetes-related complications. I was jolted out of sleep and I was hospitalized with uncontrolled diabetes and depression.

A few days after I was discharged from hospital, I had an unstoppable urge to learn all I could about Diabetes: epidemiology, predisposing factors, types of diabetes, treatment, complications, all of it.

As I continued to work as a Consultant Anaesthesiologist, I became more aware of the scourge of Diabetes. The morbidity and mortality in the hospital Outpatient Clinics, Surgical, Medical, Pediatric, Obstetric and Gynecological, Renal wards and ICU.

What about the undiagnosed diabetics? Why was diabetes becoming the biggest epidemic and one of the largest global challenges of the 21st century? Knowledge about diabetes has grown over the years! Great advances have been made in its pathophysiological, pharmacological and non-pharmacological management, but the epidemiology of diabetes is worrying. In 2015, 1 in every

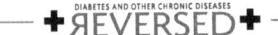
11 individuals was diagnosed with diabetes. Out of 415 million diabetics worldwide, 46.5% or 193 million people have undiagnosed diabetes. 80% of diabetics are in Low and Middle-income Countries. *5 million annual deaths worldwide are due to diabetes.*

KEY TAKEAWAYS:

- *The psychological impact of diabetes is often overlooked.*
- *Despite the advancement in diagnosis and management of diabetes, the spread of diabetes is worrying*

Out of 415 million diabetics worldwide,
46.5% or 193 million people have
undiagnosed diabetes.

CHAPTER TWO

HISTORY OF DIABETES MELLITUS (DM)

*R*ita Lakhtakia: The History of DM (2)Outlines the origins, symptoms, and signs of the disease from B.C. to the present day. It outlines the Pathophysiology through experimentation, identification of the cells which produce what came to be known as Insulin by the Pancreas, the discovery of insulin, progress in testing and treatment of diabetes.

The disease characterized by the *"too great emptying of urine"* described in Egyptian manuscripts dates back to 1500BC. Indian Physicians called it *Madhumeha (honey urine)* because it attracted ants (400-500AD).

In 1st Century AD, Areteus the Cappadocian coined the word Diabetes (*Siphon*). The term Mellitus was coined by John Rollo in 1789. The pancreas was identified as the body organ that produces Insulin in 1909. In the Pre-insulin era, calorie restriction diet and exercise were the hallmark of treatment of diabetes and it was a rare disease.

In diabetes before and after insulin: Allan F. L. (3) "The status of treatment of diabetes before insulin portrays a picture of a hopeless situation of patients succumbing to diabetic gangrene and coma and how the first human treatment of a young diabetic with Pancreatic Extract saved him in 1922.

In the Pre-insulin days, the average doctor felt hopeless in the treatment of diabetes, opium and personal hygiene were used as treatment in the 1800's. Diabetes was rare in those days: for example, records of cases of Diabetes Mellitus in the Massachusetts General Hospital USA from 1824-1898 in the medical wards were only 172.

Before the discovery of the Pancreatic Extract in 1921, other researchers had contributed immensely. Oral hypoglycemic agents were to come later but after Insulin discovery, Insulin remains a predominantly important factor in diabetes management.

In *Diabetes mellitus: "A complete ancient and modern historical perspective"*by DR Chukwuemeka Nwaneri (4) gives a detailed discussion of diabetes history covering different eras.

a) Ancient time (Era of recognition of disease in Egypt and Greece etc. in BC.)
b) First Century (Era of description of causes of DM in Greece and China)
c) Sixteen to Eighteenth century (Era of clinical diagnosis)
d) Eighteenth to Nineteenth Century (Era of biochemical and pathological differentiations)
e) Nineteenth to Twentieth-century (Era of insulin development)
   - Discovery of glucometers
   - New Insulins and insulin pumps
   - Oral glycemic control drugs
   - Bariatric surgery
f) Twenty-First Century (Era of millennium developments)
   - Newer insulins
   - Investigations: HbA1c
   - Newer oral glycemic control medications e.g. Liraglutide

In 1980, the first human insulin (Humulin) was manufactured (5). Insulin syringes and insulin pumps, inhaled insulin and oral sprays later followed. *Pancreatic transplantation was done in 1966 (6).*

From the history of diabetes, we have made great strides in understanding and management of Diabetes. Why is it projected to be the 7th leading cause of death worldwide in 2030? *International Diabetes Federation (IDF)(7),* diabetes *Atlas* 2015 shows in detail the global burden of Diabetes, estimated number of people with diabetes worldwide and per region in 2015, and as a growing epidemic with diabetes and impaired glucose tolerance projections in 2040.

KEY TAKEAWAYS:
- *Diabetes Mellitus was a rare disease.*
- *The discovery of insulin changed the management of Diabetes Mellitus and greatly improved the quality of life for patients, especially for type-1 diabetes.*

CHAPTER THREE

DIABETES IS NOT A CHRONIC PROGRESSIVE DISEASE!

In 2012 I started working as a General Practitioner and Consultant Anesthesiologist in a private hospital in the small urban town where I was born and brought up. It didn't take me long to realize that diabetes and its complications was not a large Cosmopolitan town problem but was equally worse in small urban areas and rural populations. The number of known diabetics locally was steadily increasing. What had changed in just one generation to cause the high diabetes prevalence?

As I continued managing my diabetes with oral hypoglycemic agents and the conventional diet, I noticed that though my blood sugars were well-managed, I was progressively developing tingling sensation and numbness of the feet and severe backache. I was developing a common complication of Diabetes Mellitus Type-2 (DMT2) called Peripheral Neuropathy (PN). I knew I was heading to a more chronic progressive disease. I researched widely, even came across unbelievable online methods of curing diabetes: boiled mango leaves, okra soaked in water overnight and just as the early remedies of diabetes included diverse and interesting prescriptions like oil of roses, dates, raw quinces, gruel jelly of vipers flesh, broken red corals and fresh flowers of blind nettles, they were not effective.

In 2015, I came across a lecture by *Sarah Hallberg: Reversing type2 diabetes starts by ignoring the guidelines: (8).* As an Obesity Specialist, she talks about Insulin Resistance as the cause of DMT2. She discusses the obese patient's frustration with ineffective doctors' advice and reveals that obesity is due to Insulin Resistance which leads to high insulin and blood glucose levels i.e. prediabetes and type-2 Diabetes.

Insulin is a fat-storing hormone leading to obesity. Dietary fats lead to mild elevation of insulin compared to a very high elevation of insulin after carbohydrate intake. Insulin resistance is a state of carbohydrate intolerance; *the minimum daily dietary carbohydrate requirement is zero*, therefore it is not an essential nutrient. Cutting dietary carbohydrates leads to a drop in blood insulin levels. Insulin Resistance is the most important cardiovascular risk factor. Low carbohydrate diets lead to a reduction or discontinuation of diabetic medications including insulin. A low carbohydrate diet is not zero carbohydrate neither is it a high protein diet.

She recommends the following food rules:
  a) If a foodstuff is said to be low fat or fat-free, do not buy
  b) Eat real food
  c) Don't eat what you don't like
  d) Eat when you are hungry

Many research trials to back low carbohydrate high fat (LCHF) diets are available. LCHF diet saves for the patient in terms of low or no medications. Diabetes is a chronic progressive disease unless we reduce dietary carbohydrates. This leads to diabetes remission/cure. *"Let food be thy medicine"*.

During this time, I came to know that the American Diabetic Association (ADA) Guidelines recommended a Low Fat, medium Protein and High Carbohydrate (LFHC) diet, which was part of the problem. I had also discovered that *'reducing dietary carbohydrates could reverse diabetes'*. It was the first time in 35years of my Medical Career to hear that DMT2 could be reversed!

I felt challenged to learn more. Was reversing DMT2 based on truth or were these baseless allegations without any scientific backing? Diabetes is said to be a chronic progressive Metabolic Disorder.

I went back to the Classification of Diabetes into the following categories:
  1. Type-1 DM (DMT1) due to autoimmune beta cell destruction, usually leading to absolute insulin deficiency. Prevalence of 7-10%.
  2. Type-2 DM (DMT2) due to progressive loss of beta-cell insulin secretion frequently on the background of Insulin Resistance.

3. Gestational DM (GDM) diabetes diagnosed in the second and third trimester of pregnancy that was not overt diabetes prior to gestation.
4. Specific types of diabetes due to other causes e.g. monogenic diabetic syndromes e.g. neonatal diabetes and maturity-onset diabetes of the young (MODY), diseases of exogenous pancreas such as Cystic fibrosis and pancreatitis, and drug or chemical induced diabetes e.g. Glucocorticoid use.
Prevalence of GDM and other types is 1-3%.

I was suffering from DMT2 because of the age at diagnosis, the response to oral hypoglycemic agents and the conventional diabetic diet. Since DM is a chronic progressive disease, 5-years after diagnosis and with good blood sugar (glycemic) control, I was having signs of lower limb nerve damage (diabetic neuropathy) and although it is said good glycemic control can slow progression of diabetic complications, I extrapolated; further development of the complications, more oral hypoglycemic agents (OHA), Insulin injections, amputations. This encouraged me to delve further into research.

Newer OHA were introduced into the medical field promising better glucose control and prevention of diabetes complications: Metformin, pioglitazone, sulphonylureas, glinides, acarbose, sitagliptin, GLP-1 receptor antagonists: Liraglutide, selective sodium-glucose transportation 2 inhibitors: Canagliflozin and newer Insulins.

In DM tissues become less insulin sensitive (insulin resistance-IR). More insulin is required to persuade adipose tissues and skeletal muscles to continue glucose uptake and utilization. Failure of this compensatory mechanism results in impaired glucose tolerance (prediabetes state) which progresses to DMT2. Insulin resistance (IR) sets in due to age, genetic factors, obesity, smoking, poor sleep, lack of exercise, pregnancy, etc.

I started exercising; cycling, walking and reduced my workload leading to a better sleep pattern.

I was still slightly obese with a body mass index (BMI) of 28 but it was proving difficult to lose weight while still adhering to the dietary guidelines, lifestyle changes, and medications.

I came across, *Treatment of Diabetes by DR Eric Westman (9)*. As an Obesity Medicine Specialist, he says that Protein is essential; the body can use fat or carbohydrate for energy. Elliot Proctor Joslin (1893), recommended treatment of a diabetic patient - Mary H., by starvation/fasting, then Low carbohydrate foods and fat were used to treat diabetes. The recommended diabetic diet in the pre-insulin era 1914-1921 was low-carbohydrate high-fat with large amounts of vegetables.

Before the discovery of insulin, a patient with type-1 diabetes would become emaciated because of the inability to store fat and loss of energy from chronic glycosuria. Despite high energy intake, no storage would occur; this was called *'starvation in the midst of plenty'* because the body would be thin despite large energy intake. Insulin replacement for insulin deficiency in type-1 diabetes allowed individuals to live.

Type-2 diabetics, however, have high insulin in the body (hyperinsulinemia) and hyperglycemia. Insulin resistance enables the body to store fat but cannot use it for energy i.e. has fat body habitus (excess fat store), starvation due to glucose swings but has constant fat storage (can't access fat). Therefore, the remedy is to reduce Insulin in type-2 diabetes. Medicines (glycemic control agents) lower glucose levels leading to hunger and excess eating of more carbohydrates. Reducing dietary carbohydrates leads to reduced postprandial glucose (hyperglycemia) and Insulin rise.

The lowest limit of dietary carbohydrate intake is zero. Studies on LCHF diets recommend less than 20 gm daily carbohydrate intakes to produce ketonuria. The total blood volume in the body has 5gm total glucose; that means less than half teaspoonful of sugar. Good carbs have a low glycemic index (GI), bad carbs have a high glycemic index. The low carb ketogenic diet reduces insulin and oral hypoglycemic agent's requirement and HbA1c. Exercise does not make a person lose weight.

Summary:
1. Instructing people to limit carbohydrate grams leads to a spontaneous reduction in caloric intake (without explicitly limiting calorie) and loss of body weight, improvement in glucose, improved fasting blood

profiles, triglycerides, HDL, total cholesterol/HDL ratio, improvement in systolic blood pressure and reduction in waist circumference.

2. A low carbohydrate diet is the preferred diet for Type-2 Diabetes and Metabolic Syndrome.

3. "Prevailing treatment by use of medications and a high carbohydrate diet was never compared to the Low Carbohydrate High-fat diet in clinical research".

Further research led me to *Insulin toxicity and how to cure Diabetes by DR Jason Fung: Nephrologist: (10).* "It is said that diabetes type-2 is a chronic progressive disease, which is caused by insulin resistance (IR), but what causes IR?"

High persistent levels of the hormone causes downregulation of its receptors; therefore Insulin causes IR, chronic physiological hyperinsulinemia leads to IR and IR leads to obesity. High insulin secretion is the primary insult. Genetics lead to increased insulin which leads to IR which leads to obesity. Insulin is produced in a versatile manner physiologically.

Conclusion:
1. Insulin causes Insulin resistance (IR)
2. IR causes hyperinsulinemia
3. IR requires a high persistent level of insulin; therefore, insulin causes diabetes.

Better glycemic control does not lead to better control of diabetic complications. Insulin treatment has toxicity; low serum Insulin is associated with low cardiovascular disease. Hyperinsulinemia leads to Atherosclerosis, Insulin causes salt and water retention, low HbA1c is a risk factor not due to hypoglycemia but due to Insulin toxicity. Insulin infusion post-myocardial infarction (MI) increases mortality. Diabetes is associated with increased cancer; metformin reduces cancer risk.

Insulin cures type-1 diabetes but causes type-2 diabetes. IR leads to increased Insulin which leads to decreased HbA1c, weight gain, increased MI, increased cancer. You can't treat hyperinsulinemia state with more Insulin. Glucose lowering e.g. Acarbose without hyperinsulinemia leads to improved cardiovascular outcomes. Decreased Insulin reduces diabetes; e.g.

1. Use drugs like metformin, not sulphonylureas
2. Bariatric surgery: surgery cures diabetes
3. A low carbohydrate diet reverses Type-2 diabetes.
4. Fasting: hunger disappears. Fasting reduces plasma insulin but blood glucose becomes stable; it maintains resting metabolic rate, improves insulin sensitivity, increases norepinephrine i.e. more energy and increases growth hormone.

Intermittent fasting is better than continuous fasting. Fasting in Mediterranean people gives better results of the diet than the diet itself. Fasting reduces diabetes, preserves lean muscle mass, and lowers triglycerides and LDL. Fasting is associated with reduced diabetes and lower coronary artery disease, therefore diabetes is curable. Lowering the insulin levels e.g. a 6-12-month intensive fasting regime cures diabetes with no use of medications".

Further research led me to *The Art and Science of low carbohydrate diet by DR Jeff Volek (11).* "The body can use glucose and fat. The obesity epidemic and diabetes type-2 is associated with Insulin Resistance (IR). IR is a type of carbohydrate intolerance; in patients with IR carbohydrate is converted by the liver to fat leading to increased blood triglyceride. A ketogenic diet requires taking equal or less than 20% of total calories from carbohydrates daily.

Ketones are hepatically energy-containing substances derived from fatty acids that provide fuel to nearly every cell in the body. Nutritional ketosis is the process of accelerating the production of ketones through the restriction of carbohydrates.

Keto-acidosis is a dangerous complication of type-1 diabetes (DMT1) or poorly controlled DMT2. Keto adaptation is the process of the body shifting from glucose to predominantly fat for fuel.

LEVEL OF KETONES	MMols/Litre
Moderate carb diet (fed state)	less than 0.1
Moderate carb diet (fasted state)	0.1-0.3
Moderate carb diet (fasting for weeks)	5-7

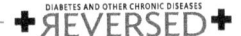

Very low carb diet (VLCD) less than 50gm/day	0.5 - 3.0
VLCD (post exercise)	1.0-5.0
Ketoacidosis (insulin insufficiency)	10 - 20+

The brain can rely on glucose and ketones; during starvation (fasting) it uses 2/3 ketones and 1/3 glucose. There is no symptom of hypoglycemia in the presence of ketones e.g. in athletes.

There are many benefits of ketones, the main ketone: beta-hydroxybutyrate (BHB) is more than a fuel, it influences gene expression.

Low carbohydrate diets are used in weight loss, reduction of cardiovascular risk factors according to many meta-analyses. There is promising research exploring the therapeutic use of ketogenic diets in DMT2, DMT1, epilepsy, obesity, Parkinson's disease, autism, migraine, Alzheimer's disease, cancer, etc. Ketogenic diets are more likely to affect global improvement in markers of Metabolic Syndrome but in 15-20% of the patients LDL increases but other markers including blood pressure and other anti-inflammatory markers decrease. Ketogenic diets decrease LDL particle sizes thus reducing cardiovascular risk. The size of LDL particles is more important than the concentration of LDL cholesterol.

There is no evidence that dietary saturated fats cause heart disease. A high carbohydrate diet leads to an increase in fatty acid composition.

Palmitoleic acid (16:1) is a marker of many diseases without high blood sugar but patients with a high level of 16:1 are at risk of developing DMT2. High carbohydrate intake leads to increased circulating saturated fatty acids especially palmitoleic acid (16:1) and exacerbates the features of insulin resistance (IR). Sustainability of the ketogenic diet is possible."

A study: ***Low carbohydrate ketogenic diet to treat type-2 diabetes: DR William Yancy et al (12)*** had a background that low carbohydrate ketogenic diet (LCKD) was effective for improving glycaemia and reducing medications in patients with type-2 diabetes (DMT2).

From an outpatient clinic, 28 overweight DMT2 participants were recruited and counseled with an initial goal of fewer than 20 grams of dietary carbohydrates

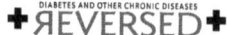
per day, while reducing diabetic medications at diet initiation. Participants returned every other week for measurements, counseling and further medication adjustments. The primary outcome was HbA1c.

Conclusion:

The LCHF diet improved glycemic control in patients with DMT2 such that medications were discontinued or reduced in most participants. Because the Low Carbohydrate Ketogenic Diet (LCKD) can be very effective at lowering blood glucose, patients on diabetic medications who use this diet should be under close medical supervision or capable of adjusting their medications.

The patients had weight loss, decreased HbA1c, serum triglycerides, and medication reductions or stoppage.

KEY TAKEAWAYS:

- *Despite well-controlled blood glucose levels using conventional medications, complications from diabetes mellitus are inevitable.*
- *Insulin causes insulin resistance (IR); IR requires a high persistent level of insulin; therefore, insulin causes diabetes.*
- *Limiting carbohydrate intake leads to a spontaneous reduction in loss of body weight, waist circumference, improved blood glucose, improved fasting blood profiles, and improvement in systolic blood pressure.*
- *Diabetes type-2 is reversible by reducing dietary carbohydrates. A low carbohydrate diet is the preferred diet for Type-2 Diabetes and Metabolic Syndrome.*

Fasting is associated with reduced diabetes and lower coronary artery disease, therefore diabetes is reversible. Lowering the insulin levels e.g. a 6-12-month intensive fasting regime reverses diabetes type-2 with no use of medications".

CHAPTER FOUR

WHAT IS WRONG WITH CONVENTIONAL DIETARY GUIDELINES

I started asking myself, what were the American Diabetic Association (ADA) Guidelines and what led to the issuance of these Guidelines? Why were the Guidelines described as faulty? Which dietary Guidelines do we follow in Kenya? I read the American Dietary Recommendations and how they had changed over time. The *American Dietary Recommendations (ADR) (13)* has been given since 1900 and is supposed to be published at least every 5 years.

1. Early food guidance 1900-1940's. 1916 first United States Department of Agriculture USDA food Guide
2. 1940's to 1970: Recommended Dietary Allowances (RDA)
3. New Direction for dietary guidelines 1970-1990s, 1977 dietary goals for the United States select committee which mainly recommended moderation of fat intake, cholesterol, and sodium.
4. Release of Food Pyramid and the Nutrition Facts Label in the 1990s
5. Fourth Edition of the Dietary Guidelines for Americans, 1995.

In 1977 the US Senate Select Committee on Nutrition and Human Needs, led by Senator George McGovern recommended (Dietary Goals) for the American people:

- Increased Carbohydrate intake 55-60% calories
- Decreased dietary fat to no more than 30% calories, etc.

The issuance of the Dietary Goals was met with a great deal of debate and controversy from both industry groups and the scientific community. These groups believed the science might not have supported the specificity of the numbers in the Dietary Goals.

"How the US Low Fat Diet Recommendations of 1977 contributed to the declining health of Americans: Julia Reedy: 2016 (14), in 1950 blood

lipoproteins were discovered, these particles HDL and LDL cholesterol were found in serum of 100 out of 104 subjects with Atherosclerosis and it was concluded that the two were directly connected to serum cholesterol role in Coronary Heart Disease (CHD) and mortality. In 1953 *Ancel Keys* (1904-2004) published an article stating that though dietary survey failed to show a connection between dietary cholesterol and serum cholesterol, controlled human studies showed that dietary fats had a direct link to blood cholesterol and Cardiovascular Disease (CVD) mortality.

Keys then cited the statistically significant discrepancies in incidence and mortality in all circulatory disease and degenerative heart disease between the US and the other Nations as the driving force behind the **Seven Countries Study** (USA, Greece, Italy, Spain, South Africa, Japan, and Finland) (SCS) piloted in 1958. Keys and his colleagues hypothesized that CHD was directly related to fat composition in the diet and serum cholesterol level, and there was a direct link between dietary saturated fats, plasma cholesterol levels, and CHD mortality rates.

American Heart Association (AHA) 1961 published a report regarding dietary fat and its relation to heart attack and stroke risk; they advised Americans to reduce fat intake, especially saturated fat, all these led to 1977 ADR and American doctors began advising dietary alterations as per the recommendations. Since then, Americans have witnessed an increase in heart disease (CVD) BMI and obesity, DMT2 and other chronic diseases.
The 2015 ADR is more comprehensive and much has been improved but more needs to be done to correct the 1977 mistakes".

Various research articles and academic lectures affirm that the 1977 US Dietary Guidelines were faulty and based on bad science e.g.

i)   *Demonization and Deception Research on saturated fats, cholesterol and heart disease by DR David Diamond (15)*

DR David Diamond first gives a story of his life: "For fifteen years his triglyceride/cholesterol was fifteen times more than the average, HDL cholesterol was low and he was at high risk of heart attack. He was advised to lower his saturated fats and commence cholesterol reduction medications

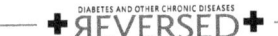
(statins). He instead decided to read widely on Nutrition and cardiovascular disease and came across Banting 1797-1878 who treated his obesity with a Low Carbohydrate diet and wrote *'the letter of opulence'*.

Many practitioners in 1950's recommended a high fat, reduced carbohydrate diet which was popularized by Atkins books in 1972. But American Heart Association recommends fat free cheese and butter etc. and low fat meat and milk.

Low fat mania started from 1955 after the death of US President Eisenhower who was a chain smoker. The story is told of *Ancel Keys, an economist and Marine Biologist and his Heart Fat hypothesis, and seven countries with high consumption of fat; he created a fake graph and became a leading researcher' of cardiovascular disease in the US. Ancel Keys advised Americans to reduce dietary fats from 40% to 15% of total calories and saturated fats: 'cooked figure', no studies*. Keys recommended Mediterranean diet, but more fat was associated with least Heart Disease e.g. France (The French Paradox).

The 1977 Senate (politicians) released Dietary Goals for USA which identified fat as the culprit for the high rate of Heart Disease in the US. This led to the Food Pyramid which is blamed for the obesity epidemic.

The 2015 US Dietary Guidelines lifted the ban on total dietary fat. The limit on total fat promoted harmful low fat foods and created cholesterol phobia. Hypercholesterolemia was alleged to predispose people to early age heart disease but there is no evidence to such. If you are 60 years and above and have high cholesterol, the chance of dying of a heart attack is 31% lower. For example, *Honolulu Heart Program: concluded that low cholesterol is associated with high mortality from stroke, Heart Disease and cancer (Jichi Medical School Cohort Study)*.

More clotting factors (fibrinogen) lead to high Heart Disease independent of cholesterol. Smoking, high blood sugar, stress, and obesity/metabolic syndrome lead to platelet activation and high risk of CVD.

Relative Risk Reduction is used cheat on drug study results e.g. Cholesterol reduction leads to no significant effect on mortality. It is alleged that Statins like

Lipitor reduces heart attacks by 36%; the actual difference is 1.1%. Atorvastatin changes the risk of heart attack by 1.1% over placebo, 98.1% atorvastatin, placebo 97%, the difference between drug and placebo is 1.1%. The ratio is 1.1%:3 this translates to 36%. Therefore relative risk reduction is legalized statistical cheating. Cretor (Jupiter Study) had a 44% Reduction in coronary events whereas Cretor v/s Placebo 1.2 %, this difference when changed to ratio and then a percentage, becomes 44%. Statins have a very small relative risk reduction but with adverse side effects; Diabetes, cancer, stroke, dementia, erectile dysfunction, rhabdomyolysis, acute renal failure, hemorrhagic stroke and liver dysfunctions.

Summary:
How statistical deception created the appearance that statins are safe and effective in primary and secondary prevention of cardiovascular disease. Junior aspirin is only advantageous in short time after first heart attack".

'Long term effects of ketogenic diet in obese subjects with high cholesterol level by Hussein Dashti et al (16) showed that a ketogenic diet leads to decrease in LDL, triglycerides and fasting blood sugar (FBS)while it increases HDL'.

In conclusion, Metabolic Syndrome is a high risk factor for obesity, cardiovascular disease and diabetes and carbohydrate restriction is most effective for its prevention.

'Dietary carbohydrate restriction as first approach in diabetes management: a critical review and Evidence Base: Nutrition 3: (2015) 1-13 Richard Feinman et al (17) confirms that dietary carbohydrate restriction reliably reduces blood glucose and elimination of medication and supports low carbohydrate diet as the first approach to treatment of diabetes type-2'.

There are twelve points of evidence supporting the use low carb diets as the first approach in treating type-2 Diabetes and the most effective adjunct to pharmacology in type-1 Diabetes

1. Hypoglycemia is the most salient feature of Diabetes. Dietary carbohydrate restriction has the greatest effect on decreasing blood sugar levels.

2. During epidemics of obesity and Type-2 Diabetes, caloric increases have almost entirely been due to increased carbohydrates.
3. Benefits of dietary carbohydrate restriction do not require weight loss.
4. Although weight loss is not required for benefit, no dietary intervention is better than carbohydrate restriction.
5. Adherence to a low carbohydrate diet in people with Type-2 Diabetes is at least as good as any other dietary interventions and is frequently significantly better.
6. Replacement of carbohydrates with proteins is generally beneficial.
7. Dietary and total saturated fats do not correlate with risk for cardiovascular disease.
8. Plasma saturated fatty acids are controlled by dietary carbohydrates more than by dietary lipids.
9. The best predictor of micro vascular and, to a least extend, macro vascular complications in patients with type-2 diabetes is glycemic control (HbA1c).
10. Dietary restriction is the most effective method (other than starvation) of reducing serum triglycerides and increasing high density lipoproteins.
11. Patients with Type-2 Diabetes on carbohydrate restricted diets reduce and frequently eliminate medications. People with type-1 usually require less insulin.
12. Intensive glucose lowering by dietary restriction has no side effects comparable to the effects of intensive pharmacological treatment.

ii) *The truth about cholesterol (18) "is a highly informative lecture by the Paleo Cardiologist Jack Wolfson.* "Cholesterol is good; it forms cell membranes, hormones: oestrogen, progesterone, cortisol, aldosterone, bile salts, and vitamin D (sun turns cholesterol to vitamin D). Breast milk has lots of cholesterol, cholesterol does not cause heart attacks e.g. Framingham Trial, AFCAP Trial.

LDL cholesterol is used to transport cholesterol, triglycerides, vitamin E, aids Coenzyme Q10 (COQ10), and prevents infections by binding to bacteria, viruses, fungi, and particles. Small LDL particles after oxidation increase cardiovascular risks.

He revisited the low-fat theory by Ancel Keys, the seven-country study and the

French paradox. Many meta-analyses have confirmed that dietary saturated fat has no association with Heart Disease.

Complications of diabetes include elevated HbA1c, an increase in the risk of cardiovascular events and cancer. Fasting Insulin levels decrease the risk of death by 31%. There is no increased risk of meat consumption (grass-fed meat). There is little evidence of an association between consumption of red and processed meat and colorectal cancer risk.

Paleolithic ketogenic diet improves glycemic control compared to a conventional diet in DMT2, increases HDL, CRP drops and decreases LDL. Genetics play a small role in Disease etiology.

There is no evidence of the advantage of statins in the prevention of cardiovascular disease.

The blood tests that really matter to a modern cardiologist, LDL Particles (a), Insulin/HbA1c, Hs-CRP/PLA2, oxidation, food sensitivity, micronutrients, MTHFR (methylation)/Homocysteine, omega 3 and vitamin D, heavy metals and autoimmune panel.

iii) *Readdressing Dietary Guidelines by DR Peter Attia (19)* starts by clarifying that calories are not just calories independent of where they come from.

The 2015 US dietary guidelines include limiting saturated fatty acid intake to less than 7% of total calories. This percentage has been going down every year. To reduce cardiovascular risk, the reduction of saturated fat calories to 5-6% is a very strong recommendation from the American Heart Association, however, there is no significant evidence to associate dietary fat with coronary heart or cardiovascular disease. He revisits DR Ancel Keys' diet-heart hypothesis and the Seven Countries study, how Keys became the most prominent Scientist/Diet adviser to the US government and the American Heart Association. The *Framingham Heart Study* found no correlation between dietary cholesterol intake and blood cholesterol.

The 1977 American Dietary Guidelines were passed due to political pressure, not scientific evidence and resulted in subsequent opposing sides.

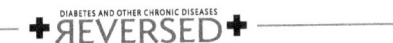
1970-1981 clinical studies showed that the amount of dietary saturated fatty acids was not significantly associated with mortality risk from CHD. Five cohort studies in the 1970's analyzed calculated LDL cholesterol which was shown to be a marginal CHD risk factor and that total cholesterol did not predict future heart disease.

In 1980 some clinical trials erroneously concluded that consensus had been reached that cholesterol causes heart disease. US Media played an important role in propagating that consensus had been reached that cholesterol, without doubt, causes heart disease.

In 2006 large clinical trials done in women showed that low dietary fat did not result in a significant reduction in the risk of CHD, stroke, diabetes or reduction in breast and colorectal cancer".

iv) *The great cholesterol myth by DR Jonny Bowden (20)*. He starts by saying, "We have been looking for the causes of diabetes, obesity, and heart disease in the wrong place. Fat does not make you fat. Low-carb high-fat diet (LCHF) can bring fat loss in obesity, but what about the saturated fat?

The American Dietary Recommendations recommend a low percentage of saturated fats. High cholesterol and heart disease are not related; cholesterol does not cause heart disease and it is not a predictor of it. 50% of ICU admissions with cardiovascular disease have normal cholesterol.

We have overprescribed cholesterol-lowering medications.

In 1990-2010, the USA has witnessed an obesity epidemic although the food pyramid is being applied and people are exercising more than ever before. China, like most countries in the world, is witnessing an increasing obesity problem; there is a failure of the low-fat diet.

Then came the Atkins diet and other low-carb high-fat diets they are good but they say, raises cholesterol levels. He revisits DR Ancel Keys Seven Countries study and the Diet-Heart Hypothesis which states that increased dietary cholesterol causes heart disease.

Clinical studies later confirmed that dietary fat is not the determinant of either hypercholesterolemia or coronary heart disease.

The *Lyon Heart study* compared people with many comorbidities on the Mediterranean diet and others on a normal diet: the plasma cholesterol did not change significantly.

LDL particle size test is the only lipid profile test that matters as a marker of cardiovascular risk. LDL-b high ratio of small particles over big particles is a high cardiovascular risk factor.
High dietary saturated fat or dietary cholesterol leads to a change in particle size; it raises the big particles and reduces the small particles which are Atherogenic.

Real promoters of heart disease are

1. Inflammation, which is due to a high carb diet and environmental toxins. Omega 3 fatty acids are anti-inflammatory while omega 6 fatty acids are pro-inflammatory. There is no minimum daily carbohydrate requirements; high dietary carbohydrate leads to hyperglycemia and high blood insulin which causes increased fat cells which produce inflammatory cytokines. Hyperglycemia leads to glycation of proteins producing advanced glycation end products (AGEs).

2. Stress and hypertension:

   Seven-point plan for reducing obesity and the risk of heart disease
   - Eat anti-inflammatory diet; low-carb high-fat diet
   - Reduce grain, starches, sugar and omega 6
   - Manage your stress
   - Exercise
   - Drink in moderation
   - Do not smoke
   - Supplement intelligently e.g. Omega 3, magnesium, COQ10, citrus bergamot extract, D-ribose, curcumin, resveratrol (dark grapes/red wine).

Summary:

1. Cholesterol does not cause heart disease nor is it a good predictor.
2. The old test for good and bad cholesterol is obsolete.
3. The conventional wisdom on saturated fats is wrong.

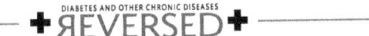
4. The demon in the diet is sugar and junk food.
5. There are nutrients that are extremely important for heart health.
6. Statin drugs have multiple and serious side effects and are being widely overused.
7. Statins have only little significant benefit in middle-aged males".

WHAT ABOUT THE SCIENTIFIC EVIDENCE?

v) *The US Dietary guidelines and scientific evidence: Nina Teicholz (21)* "Reminds us that we do follow the dietary guidelines; we eat more fruit and vegetables, whole grains, lean meat, and low-fat dairy and avoid saturated fats. The guidelines affect feeding programs for infants, schools, military, medical school curriculum; our supermarkets are full of low fat processed food products. Americans have followed the guidelines but even with more exercise, obesity has increased, so where is the science? *The guidelines are out of touch with science.*

The Mediterranean diet which was recommended for the prevention of cardiovascular disease was retracted as there was only a 0.2% difference between the diet and the normal US diet. The DASH diet trials were very short; there was no significant difference to support the vegetarian diet.

There was no evidence of any relationship between these dietary patterns and the risk of cardiovascular disease, obesity and Diabetes Type-2.

More recent rigorous Evidence for USDA-HHS dietary patterns shows that 74 trials have been done for a low carbohydrate pattern, 2 for the Mediterranean diet, DASH diet 5, and vegetarian diet 0. There are many long duration and evidence trials for a low carb diet. Low carb diets should be the gold standard for dietary guidelines.

Low-fat trials e.g. Women Health Initiative Multicenter NHS funded trial on nearly 4900 women for 8 years found that the low-fat diet did not help obesity, cardiovascular disease or any type of cancer.

Boeing trials on 1230 men and women tested on the USDA diet found no benefit, weight loss, blood sugar control (diabetes) and mild outcomes on heart disease

(LDL-C dropped but so did HDL-C and triglycerides went up) *that is why the low-fat diet is no longer officially recommended.*

A low-fat diet is ineffective and reducing total fat and replacing it with carbohydrates does not lower cardiovascular disease risk and may even worsen heart disease risk since such diets are generally associated with dyslipidemia (this is part of American dietary committee 2015).

Clinical trials on saturated fats show that reduction in saturated fat intake for prevention of cardiovascular disease had no significant effects in reducing saturated fats on all-cause mortality, cardiovascular disease mortality, events or stroke.

All evidence for the diets DASH, vegetarian and Mediterranean is epidemiological and not based on clinical trial evidence.

Conclusion:
Offer low carbohydrate diets as a viable option for fighting chronic diseases: offer a meaningful diversity of diets; make the diets nutritionally sufficient with nutrients coming from whole foods not artificially fortified refined grains; stop recommending "lower is better on salt".

Low carb diets have to be reviewed in the USDA 2020 guidelines".

vi) *Challenging conventional guidelines: The brief story behind the writing of LORE: Prof Tim Noakes (22)* "He starts by highlighting the post-exercise ketosis he was getting into in 1980. He was Insulin Resistant at 28 years though a marathoner. He and his friend had Insulin Resistance/Hyperinsulinemia despite youth and marathon training; they improved on a low-carb high-fat diet. They would develop diabetes type-2 with time as they continued eating a high carbohydrate diet; he came across the DR Atkins diet book and started practicing a low carb diet, and his diabetes went into remission.

In 2013 some people known to him reversed their diabetes with a low-carb high-fat diet. This prompted him to write the Book: *'The Real Meal Revolution'* which revolutionized the Banting diet in South Africa. He faced academic mobbing; his famous tweet led to the famous Prof Noakes Trial. Health Professions Council of

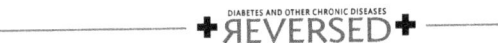
South Africa (HPCSA) conferred charges against him; the dieticians were unhappy with the fact that he was promoting a low carb high-fat diet.

The Noakes trial became the 'trial of the century' described in detail in the Book *'Lore of Nutrition'*. The 1977 US dietary guidelines is the worst thing that ever happened in Clinical Medicine".

vii) *Diet and cardiovascular disease: Message from PURE STUDY by DR Andrew Mente (23)* starts with "Diet-Heart Hypothesis: conventional wisdom that total fat, saturated fat lead to increased serum total cholesterol and LDL cholesterol which leads to coronary heart disease.

PURE is a global study that shows saturated fats lead to high cholesterol (LDL-C) and low total cholesterol/HDL (TC/HDL), and low APO-A/APOB ratio which is the strongest marker of cardiovascular risk. Higher carbohydrate intake is associated with low LDL-C, HDL-C, high TC/HDL-C, and high APO-A/APO-B ratio; higher cardiovascular risk.

Meta-analyses show no advantage of replacing saturated fats with polyunsaturated fats. The use of saturated fats showed no significant difference in various health outcomes including mortality in CVD and DMT2. Association of fats and carbohydrates intake with cardiovascular disease and mortality in 18 countries over five continents (PURE): a prospective cohort study: showed high carb intake is associated with increased mortality, higher protein intake is associated with decreased mortality, higher fat intake is associated with a lower risk of cardiovascular mortality. Higher fat intake is associated with lower risk of non-cardiovascular death. Therefore, it shows the protective effects of fats.

Fruit/vegetables and legumes were associated with a lower risk of mortality and major CVD events.

Summary:
1. A high carb diet (more than 50-55%E i.e. Total Energy requirement in calories) is associated with a higher risk of mortality.
2. Fats including saturated and unsaturated are associated with a lower risk of mortality.

3. There is no association between total fat, types of fats and cardiovascular events.
4. Current advice to limit total fat to less than 30% E and saturated fat less than 10% E are not supported by this global study.

Conclusion:

Food and health: Eat more fruit, vegetables, nuts, legumes, dairy, and meats. Eat less refined grains and sugar, processed meats, and sweetened drinks. Avoid industrial trans fats.

Salt: Central hypothesis.

Salt (sodium) intake causes high blood pressure which causes heart attack, stroke, and death-assumes that sodium has no other effects on biological systems. WHO AHA guidelines:

General recommendations: consume less than 2-2.4gm equivalent to 1 teaspoonful daily

FSA1 less than 2.4gm per day

High-risk candidates: Less than .5gm per day=0.7 teaspoonful per day

A general population study on the relationship between salt and mean blood pressure finds weak or no relationship.

In DASH and PURE Trial regardless of normal B/P low sodium causes high cardiovascular risk. Low sodium has an adverse effect on cardiovascular biomarkers e.g. renin, aldosterone, epinephrine, norepinephrine, triglycerides or increased CVD risk.

High sodium (more than 5gm per day) is associated with increased risk of stroke e.g. China

Potassium is beneficial.

Summary:

Sodium intake of more than 5gm per day is associated with higher CVD and deaths.
Such high levels of sodium are seen mainly in China and less common in other countries.

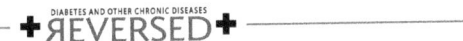

Low sodium intake is associated with higher mortality and CVD in individuals and persists after adjustment for confounders and control of reverse causality. Potassium is associated with a lower risk of CVD and deaths".

viii) Nutritional nuggets to combat conventional dietary advice/guidelines: challenging beliefs by Zoe Hercombe (24)

It challenges the following seven beliefs

1. 1lb = 3500 calories
2. The Calorie formula: A deficit of 1500 calories will produce a loss of 1lb of fat
3. Animal fat is saturated and plant fat is unsaturated
4. Saturated fat causes CHD
5. Cholesterol causes CVD
6. Whole grains are healthy
7. We must get our 5-a-day

Explanation of the above challenges:

1. Calorie formula: to lose 1lb of fat- 1lb fat contains 3500 calories, so to lose 1lb a week you need to eat 500 fewer calories a day (British Dietician Association BDA).
   - 1lb does not equal 3500 calories.
2. A deficit of 3500 calories will not lead to a loss of 1lb fat. The formula comes from where? 'Diet and Health' Lulu Hunt Peter (1918). Or British Health Authorities 2009.
   - It is not known where the formula came from but a deficit of 3500 calories will not produce a loss of 1lb of fat.
3. Animal fat is not saturated and plant fat is not unsaturated.
   - Milk has more unsaturated than saturated fats

	Meat	Eggs	Fish	Lard	Nuts	Olive oil	Milk
Total Fat	7	10	14	100	51	100	1
Unsaturated Fat	2.1	3.1	3.3	39	3.9	14	0.6

a)   Saturated fats (most stable fat)
b)   Monounsaturated fats
c)   Polyunsaturated fats

All foods that contain fat contain all three fats, there are no exceptions: meat, fish, eggs, dairy, nuts and seeds, olives and avocados. Only dairy products have more saturated than unsaturated fat not that any real fat is better or worse than any other.

1. Saturated fat causes CVD; *saturated fat does not cause CHD.*
   Epidemiology: No association for CVD or CHD.
   Random Control Test (RCTs) (pre-1983) showed no association with CHD, No RCTs had tested the 1977 guidelines. RCTs to date show no association with CHD. RCT evidence does not support the current dietary guidelines.

2. *Cholesterol does not cause CVD,* the higher the cholesterol the lower the deaths from CVD.

3. Whole grains are healthy-Really? Liver is the healthiest food.

4. Five a day is a fairy tale: it's not evidence-based.

Summary:
   1. Calorie formula: 1lb is not equal to 3500 calories
   2. Calorie formula: A deficit of 3500 will not produce a loss of 1lb of fat
   3. Animal fat is not saturated; Plant fat is not unsaturated
   4. Saturated fat is INVERSELY associated with CHD
   5. Cholesterol is INVERSELY associated with CVD.
   6. Whole grains are nowhere as healthy as animal foods
   7. 5-a-day is a myth, not a nugget.

Conventional medical practices are universal and it is not surprising that Kenyan dietary guidelines are influenced by the USA dietary guidelines of 1977 which recommend a food pyramid of low fat, medium protein, and high carbohydrate diet. Saturated fats are said to cause heart disease; traditional ghee butter and lard are discouraged while factory-made vegetable oils encouraged.

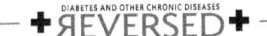
ix) Vegetable oils, the Unknown Story: Nina Teicholz (25) "Vegetable oils are not made from vegetables; they are made from beans and seeds e.g. Soybean oil, they should be called seed oils. Natural oils are tallow, suet, lard, butter, palm oil, etc. Oils were used as lubricants for machinery during the Industrial Revolution e.g. from whales and later from cottonseed.

Fats are saturated, monounsaturated and polyunsaturated. Oils were made stable by the process of hydrogenation. In 1911, vegetable and synthetic oils from cottonseed entered the food industry as human food. Commercial products like Crisco and margarine replaced dairy butter.

Vegetable oils were cheaper and it was a sign of opulence. In 1948 stable vegetable cooking oils were manufactured.

In 1961 the American Heart Association (AHA) recommended polyunsaturated oils to prevent heart disease.

Coupled with Ancel Keys diet fat heart hypothesis, Proctor and Gamble makers of Crisco became very wealthy; vegetable oils were marketed for the prevention of high cholesterol and heart disease.

Diet-Heart Hypothesis has been disapproved; there is no effect of saturated fats on CVD or total mortality. Studies on Elderly Veterans' Home in Los Angeles where Soybean oil, corn oil, sunflower, and cottonseed oils had replaced animal fats showed that they died of cancer, gallstones, stroke, and liver cirrhosis although cholesterol was lowered by vegetable oils.

Natural, stable unsaturated fats are like palm oil and coconut.

In 1980, US dietary guidelines advised the replacement of saturated fats with polyunsaturated vegetable oils, they are very cheap and became the backbone of the food industry. Advocacy groups were campaigning against natural unsaturated fats.

Trans Fats were banned and replaced with genetically modified soybean oil and interesterified oils.

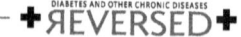
Vegetable oils are cheap but they have pro-inflammatory omega 6 and when heated produce toxic oxidation products for example aldehydes which are cancer biomarkers. Olive oil is monounsaturated and is stable when not heated.

Summary:
> Avoid polyunsaturated oils and for salad dressing use olive oil. For cooking use saturated fats e.g. lard. Avoid fried food in restaurants. 'Canola is still polyunsaturated oil'."

x) Vegetable oils: The Untold Story and the US dietary guidelines by Nina Teicholz (26) "Polyunsaturated vegetable oils are corn, cottonseed, soybean, peanut oil, safflower and canola oils.

In 2000-2015 US Dietary Guidelines recommended oils are soybean, corn oil, safflower oil, and olive oil. We have increased the consumption of these oils. Natural oils were lard, butter, and tallow. Oils from whales were for the lubrication of machinery.

From cottonseed, hydrogenation created vegetable oil (Crisco).

In 1961, saturated fats were said to be associated with heart disease but randomized clinical trials in the '60s and '70s showed no effect of saturated fats on cardiovascular mortality.

1980 Los Angeles veteran trials showed increased death rates due to cancer, although blood cholesterol levels were lowered by vegetable oils. Heating of polyunsaturated oils could have led to toxic oxidation products e.g. aldehydes which could have led to increased cancer mortality.

The dietary guidelines are out of step with science considering the oils they are recommending.

The USA Dietary Guidelines are said to have led to the global epidemic of obesity, diabetes and other metabolic disorders have resulted. The demonization of cholesterol in the multibillion lipid-lowering drugs industry: these drugs are statins and non-statins prescribed to lower the cardiovascular risk associated with high cholesterol. "But are we chasing the rat leaving the elephant in the room"?

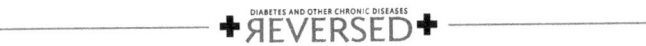

xi) *Sense and nonsense in the war of saturated fats: DR David Diamond (27)*
"He was diagnosed with Familial Hypertriglyceridemia which is associated with 15 times risk of heart disease, he was mildly obese and a low-fat diet could not improve his lipid profile. He read about the connection between carbohydrate intolerance and lipidemia and how William Banting cured his obesity with a low-carb high-fat diet.

In 1953 a high-fat diet was being recommended for obesity and in 1957 a low-carb high-fat diet was recommended for the treatment of obesity.

In 1972 the Atkins diet which was recommending a reduction of dietary carbohydrate was introduced.

Research trials on ketogenic diets had the following effect on biomarkers:
- HDL increase,
- Triglyceride/LDL ratio
- A decrease in blood sugar

Interim summary:
1. Reduced carbohydrate diets have been recognized as safe and effective in the treatment of obesity since 1863. High caliber research has shown that targeted carbohydrate reduction improves risk biomarkers (risk factors) for heart disease and DMT2 (metabolic syndrome).

2. History of increase in heart attacks in the USA: Death of Eisenhower due to heart attack, DR Ancel Keys diet Heart Hypothesis, and his seven countries study in 1961 made Ancel Keys a USA expert in Nutrition and Heart Disease. Ancel Keys came up with the idea of the Mediterranean diet. Then Politicians passed the 1977 American dietary guidelines and the Food Pyramid, this led to high carbohydrate fast foods outlets and high carbohydrate soft drinks which have contributed to the Obesity Epidemic.

Later analysis of DR Keys' findings showed there was no relationship between dietary fat and heart disease and there is no connection between egg consumption and heart disease.

High dietary fat communities like the Inuits (Eskimos) and the Maasais have a very low incidence of heart disease, France has high dietary fat consumption but low incidence of heart disease and obesity *(The French Paradox)*.

Studies that show meat-eaters have high cardiovascular mortality don't appreciate that they are more likely to be smokers, overweight and sedentary. Adding fat to the diet increases nutrient absorption e.g. beta carotenes.

Saturated fats are not associated with cardiovascular disease. There is no evidence to support the original dietary guidelines demonizing saturated fats *(Zoe Hercombe 2015)*

Summary:
- Intake of total fat was not significantly associated with coronary events (heart attacks) or mortality.
- Intake of saturated fats (animal fats) was not significantly associated with coronary events or mortality.
- Fatal heart disease was not reduced by low-fat diets or by replacing saturated (animal) fats with polyunsaturated (vegetable) fats.

In 2015 Dietary Guidelines lifted the ban on total dietary fat but saturated fat is still demonized. New dietary guidelines urge limiting added sugar and saturated fat.

There is also a challenge in conveying accurate information to the public in peer-reviewed journals. *'A generation of citizens has grown up since the Diet-Heart Hypothesis was launched as official dogma by Ancel Keys. They have been misled by the greatest scientific deception of our times: The notion that consumption of animal fat causes heart disease'. Coronary Heart Disease: Doing the Wrong things: Nutrition Today July 1985: Prof George Mann"*.

xii) *Too much medicine and great statin con: DR Aseem Maholtra (Interventional Cardiologist) (28),* "The system has become very corrupt and doctors can no longer practice honest medicine. Evidence-based medicine is the cornerstone but we have misinformed doctors because of biased research reporting in medical journals, patient pamphlets, media reporting, defensive medicine, and medical curriculum:

1. Financial conflicts of interest and culture to do more investigations and procedures unnecessarily e.g. too much angiography. More informed consent can reduce potential harms. More medicine is not better; more Medical Care in the USA does not translate to better health. Too much Medicine is harmful and wasteful. Are the procedures necessary, do they change the quality of life?

2. Doctors' understanding of health statistics is a risk factor for misinformation. 25% risk reduction of mammogram means you screen 2500 women to save one life. Misleading health statistics e.g. Relative risk reduction (RRR) and absolute risk reduction (ARR). Most journals report RRR. The risk of stopping statin medications is 1:10000 which is virtually zero. Statins do not prevent death or serious illness, there is 1:40 chance that taking statins for 5 years will prevent one fatal heart attack but there is 1:100 chance of developing diabetes. 1:5 patients taking statins will have serious unacceptable side effects; muscle pains. The statin controversy is made more complicated by the unavailability of professional data. There is no proven mortality after stopping the use of statins, neither any justification in the use of statins in low-risk people. In the illusion of innovation, doctors collude with the pharmaceutical industry for financial gain. Most of the new drugs are not innovative; it is no longer possible to trust most of the research trial results. The Statin Usage Survey (Statin usage.com) showed that:

    a) Nearly 75% of the new users discontinue statins within a year of prescription.

    b) Side effects were the leading reason why patients stopped taking statins.
       To prevent myocardial infarction, statins have very small significance; aspirin will not reduce the risk. Mediterranean diet and stent have nearly the same chance.
       There is no scientific proof that if you can't exercise or take the right diet then take a statin.
       The major problem contributing to heart disease is diet 34.6%, smoking 6.5%, alcohol 5.5% and exercise lack 3.1%".

xiii) *Statin Wars: Have we been misled by the evidence?* **DR Marianne Demasi (29)** "Statins are the most globally prescribed cholesterol-lowering drugs. Lipitor is the most profitable drug in the history of medicine; sales in the USA are $1 Trillion by 2020. The suggested indications are:

1. High-risk people,
2. Everyone with 50 years even with normal cholesterol,
3. Pediatric statins,
4. Condiments in fast-food outlets
5. Putting in public drinking water.

The proponents state that statins are most important in preventing heart disease, the skeptic's state that statins are largely unnecessary. Statinization of the population can be achieved by lowering the level of cholesterol. There is industry bias because manufacturers fund the statin trials.

Raw data on statin side effects are kept secret; data secrecy and contestability of science bring lack of transparency in science resulting in minimizing harms in trials, exaggerating statistics e.g. reporting relative risk reduction (RRR) of Lipitor of 36% instead of absolute risk reduction (ARR) of 1%, silencing the dissenters by writing review articles and using the media, discrediting dissenters and censorship from interested groups or a scare campaign e.g. making extrapolations on the effects of statin drugs".

KEY TAKEAWAYS:

- *High and Low salt intake is associated with high cardiovascular disease and deaths.*
- *Vegetable oils are NOT made from vegetables. They are cheap, pro-inflamatory and might not be safe.*
- *Statins don't prevent death or serious illnesses and have serious side effects.*
- *The 1977 US dietary guidelines have led to increase in heart disease, obesity e.t.c.*
- *Cholesterol reduction leads to no significant reduction on CVD mortality.*

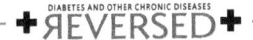
- *There is no correlation between dietary cholesterol intake and blood cholesterol*
- *High cholesterol and heart disease are not related.*
- *LDL particle size is an important marker of cardiovascular risk.*
- *Saturated fats are not associated with high CVD mortality.*
- *Consumption of animal fat does not cause heart disease.*
- *Statistics are used to falsely show the effectiveness of statins.*
- *Low-Fat diets are no longer officially recommended*

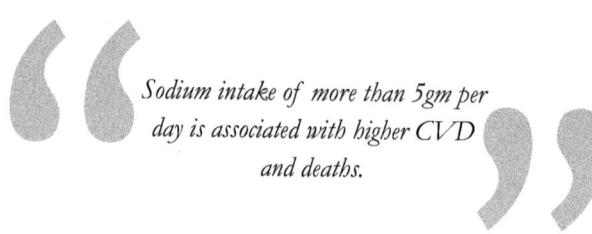

Sodium intake of more than 5gm per day is associated with higher CVD and deaths.

CHAPTER FIVE

GLYCEMIC INDEX AND GLYCEMIC LOAD

What does Nutrition have to do with Diabetes Mellitus (DM)? *Let's go back to the basics.* DM is caused by inadequate insulin secretion and or defects in Insulin action leading to Insulin resistance. Insulin is a hormone secreted by the pancreatic beta cells. Inadequate Insulin production and/or resistance cause alterations in protein, lipid, and carbohydrate metabolism and there is decreased glucose uptake and utilization by adipose tissues and skeletal muscles leading to increased blood glucose (Diabetes Mellitus).

The foods we eat (macronutrients) are mainly classified as fat, protein, and carbohydrates. By studying the Glycemic Index (GI), Glycemic Load (GL) and Insulin Index (II) of carbohydrates we can know how various carbohydrates affect Insulin production *"The international table of glycemic index and glycemic load (GL) control value 2012 (30)* covers global foods and very narrowly covers popular and staple Kenyan and specifically African foods.

Foods with high GI produce a higher peak in postprandial blood glucose and a greater overall blood glucose response during the first two hours after consumption than foods with a low GI; the higher the GI, the higher the expected elevation in blood glucose and Insulin. After digestion and absorption, fats cause little increase in blood glucose, proteins cause moderate while carbohydrates result in high blood glucose and insulin levels.

Glycemic index (GI) ranks carbohydrate foods from 0-100, i.e. High GI more than 70, Medium GI is 56-69 and low GI less than 55.

- Low GI foods (with GI less than 55) are cereals and pulses:
    - Parboiled rice, barley, green peas, lentils, kidney beans, soybeans, all dhal, and all legumes,
    - Milk and milk products: Milk, curd, cheese, etc.
    - Vegetables: all vegetables grown above the ground and underground vegetables like carrots and turnips
    - Fruits: apples, plum, pawpaw, guava,

- Medium GI foods (GI 55-69)
    - Cereals: whole wheat, basmati rice, semolina roasted, brown rice, and oatmeal
    - Vegetables and fruits: Mango, pomegranate, custard apple, banana, pineapple, black grapes, beetroot, and raisins.
- High GI foods (70-100)
    - Rice, potatoes, corn flakes, sugar, rice products, white bread.

Most of our foods are carbohydrates with high to medium GI, for example, wheat, rice, corn/maize, millet, cassava, and sweet potatoes and potatoes. This has been confirmed by studies done in Western Kenya: *Glycemic responses to stiff porridge (ugali) meals consumed in Western Kenya: Rebecca A Abere et al: (31)* "This is the first scientific research on GI of "*ugali*" widely consumed in Kenya and shows that high GI of ugali can be reduced by consuming it with vegetables.

Glycemic index of cassava and sweet potatoes consumed in Western Kenya: Rebecca A. Abere et al (32): The GI and GL of cassava and sweet potatoes are analyzed. Both have high GL while sweet potatoes have moderate GI.

An investigation on the glycemic Index of local foods and use in the Management of Diabetes Mellitus: Waudo et al, (33). This is a very comprehensive study of locally available foodstuffs;" the foods with very high GI were sweet potatoes, maize, and beans, followed by rice and beans, maize, millet, sorghum, and sweet potatoes recorded average GI while rice and green bananas recorded low GI". Generally, factory processed foods have a high GI. A meal of sweet potatoes and millet porridge recorded the highest glycemic index 124.11, followed by maize and beans recorded a GI of 63, rice and beans GI 63.87".

Some of these foodstuffs have high GI which is not recommended, even in conventional diabetes management.

Consuming high GI foods by increasing blood glucose levels leads to hyperinsulinemia state which is now recognized as the cause of metabolic syndrome with its associated chronic diseases e.g. DMT2, hypertension, obesity, hyperlipidemias, coronary heart disease, etc.

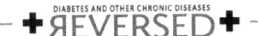
Is there a significant difference between white rice and brown rice, white wheat flour and brown wheat flour?

Does the fermentation of carbohydrates lower the GI? (34) Fermentation and germination improve the nutritional value of cereals and legumes through activation of endogenous enzymes: Smith G. Nkhata et al. Fermentation process significantly changes the nutritional value of foods by reducing antinutrients, lowering GI, etc.

The Kenya Medical Guidelines for Management of DMT2 Second Edition 2018 (35) "It is very comprehensive and informative. The Conventional Dietary Guidelines are recommended:
- Carbohydrate 45-60% of total energy intake (TEI)
- Protein 15-20% of TEI
- Fat less than 35% of TEI; saturated fats should be less than 7%, most of the fat should be unsaturated (i.e. vegetable oils).

Many scientific studies, however, have confirmed that saturated fat does not cause heart disease or obesity. The fat found in coronary heart disease is mainly polyunsaturated fat from 'healthy' vegetable oils (26)

Sugar and high carbohydrate intake increases the risk of heart disease.

Saturated fat is not dangerous: DR Paul Mason (36). The 1977 US Dietary Guidelines recommended a reduction in saturated fat. This has also been advocated in Australian Guidelines (1979-2013) but there has never been a scientific evaluation of the recommendations. Where the evidence base was unlikely to have changed substantially (e.g. the relationship between intake of foods high in saturated fats and increased risk of high serum cholesterol) additional review was not conducted. Many Meta-analytic research findings were not considered during the development of current guidelines. Research published after 2013 shows that saturated fats are not associated with CVD and/or cause mortality.

Is it harmful to reduce saturated fats? The most expensive diet study ever performed found increased harm from low-fat diets i.e. Low Fat Dietary Pattern and Risk of Cardiovascular disease Randomized Trial showed a reduction of saturated fats leads to significant mortality in some women.

Cholesterol is NOT dangerous. 75% of cholesterol is made by the body and has many physiological uses. Fat is **not** soluble in blood. Lipoproteins of different sizes transport fat in circulation e.g. HDL and LDL. LDL 1-2 is non-oxidized, LDL 3-7 are oxidized, saturated fat increases cholesterol. Carbohydrates make LDL bad. Glycated LDL cannot be taken by the liver. In atherosclerosis, increased circulating LDL particles are not taken up by the liver but are taken up by macrophages in blood vessel walls. Elevated blood glucose and increased insulin increase LDL glycation thus increasing the risk of heart disease.

What effects do statins have on lifespan? After taking statins for 5 years and with a previous history of heart disease lifespan will be increased by 5.2 days, and if there's no history of heart disease lifespan will be increased by 3.2 days!

Vegetable oils have more omega 6 and are therefore inflammatory. Eicosanoids are derived from omega 3 or omega 6 fats and maintenance of their ratios is important.

Saturated fats help to make cholesterol and cholesterol is important in the making of cell membranes, healing mechanisms (inflammation), organs (brain), emotional health, etc. ***Cholesterol when to worry: Prof Sikaris (37).*** "Cholesterol is used to make bile which helps to absorb fat, stiffens cell membranes, is a precursor for vitamin D and all sex hormones e.g. testosterone.

Ancel Keys Lipid Hypothesis stated that the higher the cholesterol or dietary saturated fat the higher the risk of heart disease. *Recent studies confirm the opposite; the higher the cholesterol the less the mortality rate.* Cholesterol is in lipoproteins from HDL, small LDL, to very large VLDL, chylomicrons. The liver makes the big particles VLDL which float in blood and gradually the triglycerides are taken off from it into the muscle tissues etc. and as they get smaller only the small LDL are left, the LDL then goes back to the liver. If LDL receptors in the liver fail LDL cholesterol will raise. Abnormalities in LDL receptors lead to LDL staying in blood for long e.g. in Diabetes. An increase in small LDL leads to cardiovascular disease.

In Familial Hypercholesterolemia, there is small LDL accumulation, therefore, giving statins improves the risk of cardiovascular disease by reducing small

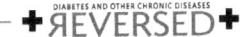
dense LDL. Only small dense LDL is related to increased cardiovascular disease risk.

Glycated and oxidized LDL are Atherogenic and therefore increase the risk of cardiovascular disease. High cholesterol leads to high HDL but Total Cholesterol (TC) can be high with a small dense LDL. High triglycerides (more than 5) are associated with high small dense LDL e.g. in diabetes. Triglyceride to HDL ratio is a better predictor of cardiovascular risk. Effective treatments decrease triglycerides which decrease small dense LDL.

Carbohydrate Restriction studies in diabetes and metabolic syndrome results in the greatest reduction of triglycerides and small dense LDL.

Summary
1. Cholesterol is good; there is not enough reason to worry.
2. LDL-C is normally good; large and buoyant is normal
3. Modified LDL is bad:
    - Small density LDL, glycated or oxidized (triglycerides more than 1.5mmol/litre)
    - APO-A or APO-B, the higher they are the higher the cardiovascular risk

When do we worry about modified LDL? We don't have to worry because Low carb high-fat diet (LCHF) reduce low-density LDL, oxidized, or glycated LDL.

Learn more about lipoprotein A and B and PCS K9.

Although it is clear that diabetes is a disease of low insulin production and/or insulin resistance leading to the inability to metabolize mainly carbohydrate adequately, our dietary guidelines still recommend a high carbohydrate, medium protein, and low-fat diet.

Are dietary carbohydrates an essential macronutrient? The human body cannot survive without fat and protein but can survive without dietary carbohydrates since the liver can make enough glucose from excess protein and energy sources from fat so long as there is enough dietary fat and protein. Of all methods of

DMT2 control, reduction of dietary carbohydrates i.e. a low carbohydrate diet is the most effective *(12)*.

As I continued researching, I came across *Nutritional Ketosis*. This is a body's metabolic shift from utilizing glucose as a source of fuel (energy) to using ketones for energy. When dietary carbohydrate intake is low, the liver converts fat into ketone bodies; these are acetone, aceto-acetone, and beta-hydroxybutyrate. Ketones are a good and safe energy source for the body. Pregnant women, babies, and normal healthy people use ketones during fasting. Ketones are a better energy source for the human brain and muscles than glucose. The levels of ketones during Nutritional Ketosis are low and safe and they are associated with normal levels of insulin and blood glucose.

In diabetic ketoacidosis (DKA) due to insulin insufficiency in DMT1 and insulin resistance (IR) in DMT2, the levels of ketones are more than 10 times higher than in nutritional ketosis. In Nutritional Ketosis blood ketone bodies is 0.5-3mg/dl or 0.05-0.29mmol/L. Blood ketones in DKA are 15-30mg/dl. Very high ketone levels are toxic to the brain leading to metabolic acidosis and can be fatal *(9)*.

KEY TAKEAWAYS:

- *Most of the processed foods have a high glycemic index.*
- *Modified LDL is bad.*
- *Most African traditional foodstuffs have lower Glycaemic Index (GI) than processed foods.*
- *Dietary carbohydrate is not an essential macronutrient*
- *Nutritional Ketosis is safe, however Diabetic Ketoacidosis (DKA) can be fatal*

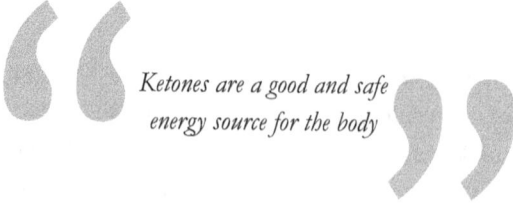

Ketones are a good and safe energy source for the body

CHAPTER SIX

NUTRITIONAL KETOSIS

*T*he art and science of Nutritional Ketosis DR Stephen Phinney (38) "followed the Atkins diet to improve his cycling performance and realized that the body becomes capable of metabolizing fats after the first four weeks. In 1980 he coined the terms 'Nutritional Ketosis' and 'Keto Adaptation'. Most people have had no teaching in Nutrition or Nutritional Ketosis. Nutritional Ketosis is a safe tool if used properly but it is not safe in people to whom it is contraindicated. The LCHF ketogenic diet should not consider low carbohydrates only but other aspects of the diet.

Ketones are made in the liver from body fat or blood lipoproteins and they are used as fuel by the brain and muscles. Ketones are gene signaling molecules in diabetes, heart disease, inflammatory bowel disease (IBD), high blood pressure, epilepsy, etc. Ketones also reduce oxidative stress.

Type-1 diabetes leads to ketoacidosis; these are high levels of ketones in the bloodstream approximately 20mg/dl. Eating a well-formulated ketogenic diet leads to ketone levels between 0.5-3mg/dl, i.e. NutritionalKetosis. One gets into nutritional ketosis by having insulin resistance in type-2 diabetes, or obesity, or by lowering daily carbohydrate intake to below 20-50gms per day, i.e. 5-10% of the daily energy intake from carbohydrates. This is not a high protein diet which will raise insulin level but moderate. The ketogenic diet is not calorie-restricted, the majority of the calories come from fat. Vegetables provide enough micronutrients, fiber, and satiety i.e. 3 to 5 servings. Every person has their own protein needs.

There are many low carbohydrate diets not necessarily ketogenic e.g. Paleo, low carbohydrate Mediterranean with intermittent fasting. These do not allow for keto-adaptation. You should measure your blood ketones to know you are keto-adapted. To apply the ketogenic diet safely, knowledgeable medical personnel and support supervision is required. Make sure you are getting all your minerals; sodium, potassium, zinc, iron, calcium which decrease during nutritional ketosis.

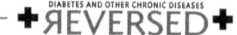
These are obtained from vegetables and bone broth, vitamins are mainly got from vegetables.

The ketogenic diet can be sustained for decades and is a disease reversing diet with many applications.

These low carbohydrate diets lead to the production of ketone bodies which are used as energy (fuel) sources instead of glucose; they are referred to as Low-carbohydrate, high-fat (ketogenic) (LCHF) diets. They are being used in reversing DMT2 and other non-communicable diseases.

Ketogenic diets and diabetes (39) DR Richard Feinman PhD: He questions; can we generalize about Metabolic Syndrome and what is its impact? What is the impact of carbohydrate restriction on diabetes management and what is the relationship between diabetes and cancer?

Clinically, Metabolic Syndrome includes at least three of the following, overweight, hyperglycemia, insulin resistance, high blood pressure, and Atherogenic dyslipidemias i.e. triglycerides, low HDL, high small and dense LDL. Is insulin resistance the common feature? All these are improved by a low carbohydrate diet.

Carbohydrate restriction targets all the markers of Metabolic Syndrome without side effects while drugs target individual markers of the Metabolic Syndrome. Diabetes is a disease of carbohydrate intolerance and dietary restriction should be the first approach in diabetes management and in Critical review and evidence based Review articles. The twelve points of evidence supporting the use of low carb diets were discussed in *(17).*

DR Westman: LCHF and diabetes theory and practice (40) starts with the history of diabetes. In 1893 Elliot proctor Joslin recommended a low carbohydrate high fat diet to diabetic patient Mary H.

Fredrick Allen used fasting then restricted carbohydrate diet, protein and fat to treat diabetes. During the Pre-insulin era, Diabetes Type-1 (DMT1) patients used to emaciate and die, then Ancel Keys came with his Fat-Heart Hypothesis and guidelines which favor medications and a high carbohydrate diet for DMT2.

Insulin treatment for Type-2 Diabetes (DMT2) does not address Insulin Resistance. Very low carbohydrate intake reduces Postprandial Glycemic/Insulin response.

Clinical studies were done in 2005; Three showed the effect of carbohydrate intake and glycemic control, Two control effectiveness and Three efficacy studies. All the studies showed that the lower the daily carbohydrate intake, the lower the mean HBA1c.

Daily carbohydrate requirements:
1. The lowest limit of carbohydrate compatible with life is zero, provided that adequate amounts of protein and fat are consumed.
2. The minimal exogenous and endogenous carbohydrates are dependent upon the brain (100-140gm glucose per day).
3. After Keto Adaptation 80% of the CNS energy can be derived from ketones leaving 20% (20-28gm) glucose per day.
4. Endogenous glucose production rate: 2-2.5gm per kg/minute to 2.8-3.6gm per kg/minute per day. In a 70kg man, this represents 210-270gm per day (Institute of Dietary reference Intakes 2008).

Studies (2006-2014) on carbohydrate restriction with a ketogenic diet (KD) and Type-2 Diabetes confirm that KD works better than low-calorie diets as evidenced by the reduction in HBA1c.

Total blood sugar is 5gm i.e. 1teaspoonful. Good carbohydrate foods have a low GI and bad carbohydrate foods have a high GI. Lowering the daily carbohydrate intake increases the chance of going into Nutritional Ketosis.

The lowest limit of carbohydrate compatible with life is zero, provided that adequate amounts of protein and fat are consumed

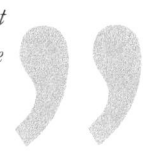

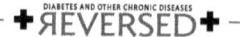
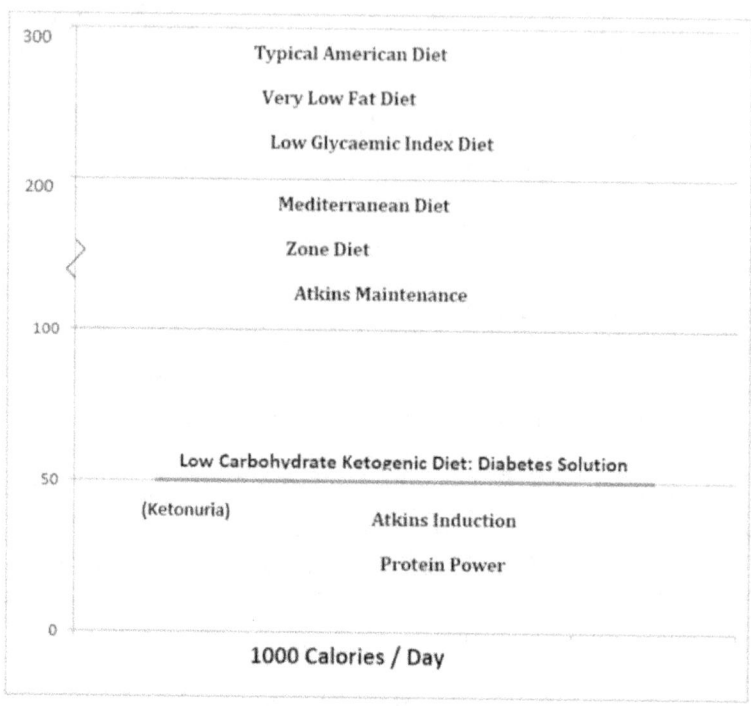

In a low carbohydrate ketogenic diet maintain dietary carbohydrate at less than 20gm per day and no counting of calories.

After starting the LCHF diet insulin dose should be reduced by half on the first day. Insulin and other glycemic medications should be reduced gradually. The ketogenic diet can lead to no hypertension, GERD, Diabetes Type-2, and a decrease in BMI without medications.

Summary:
1. Instructing patients to restrict carbohydrate grams leads to a spontaneous reduction in caloric intake (without explicitly limiting calories) and body weight, improvements in glucose, fasting serum lipid profiles (triglycerides, HDL, total cholesterol/HDL ratio), improvement in systolic blood pressure, and reduction in waist circumference.

2. A Low Carb is the preferred diet for Metabolic Syndrome and Type-2 Diabetes.

3. The prevailing treatment with medications and a high carb diet was never compared to the low-carb high-fat diet (LCHF) in clinical research.

Other than LCHF diets to reverse DMT2; what other non-conventional methods are used alone or with LCHF:

a) **Exercise**

Although it is known to be ineffective, exercise and Conventional High Carbohydrate diets are recommended in Obesity and associated DMT2.

Fasting, autophagy and exercise Mike Mutzel (41) Autophagy is the process of maintenance of the proteome by balancing synthesis and recycling of intracellular proteins; this process is related to aging and therefore increased autophagy delays aging and promotes longevity.

Most of autophagy in humans is enhanced by exercise (not by fasting as often thought). More exercise leads to more Insulin sensitivity. Autophagy was first described in 1859, mTor inhibits autophagy. Autophagy leads to stem cell activation. There are activators e.g. hormones and inhibitors. Imbalance of autophagy leads to diseases e.g. Crohn's disease.

After exercise, autophagy repairs the skeletal muscles.

Exercise-induced autophagy leads to improvement in neurodegenerative diseases e.g. Alzheimer's disease.

Endurance exercises lead to increased autophagy. Calorie restriction diet, low protein diet, and exercise increase autophagy. Some pharmacological drugs and mushrooms enhance autophagy.

b) **Intermittent fasting** is said to reduce insulin levels making it easy for the body to use stored fat, lowering blood sugar, blood pressure, and inflammatory markers and promotes longevity.

Applications of intermittent fasting in medicine (42): DR Jason Fung (Nephrologist) Diabetes type-2 is not a chronic progressive disease; it is a disease of hyperinsulinemia due to Insulin resistance (IR) which can be treated with a low carbohydrate ketogenic diet and or intermittent fasting (IF). Individual fasting protocols are applied depending on different goals; obesity/weight loss, autophagy, cancer, DMT2 e.g. a 24 hour fast. The adjustment of Insulin and other hypoglycemic medications should start before commencing the fast in DMT2 patients.

The following baseline blood tests should be done prior to the fast; HBA1c, fasting blood sugar (FBS), Vitamin D and Iron. The regularity of these tests is dependent on the disease. Coffee, MCT oil, green tea, bone broth, citrus fruit juices, and ginger can be consumed during the fast. Green tea increases metabolic rate and reduces hunger. IF reduces mTor, MPK and other growth pathways leading to a reduction in tumor growth, Alzheimer's disease improvement, increase in longevity by increasing autophagy and PCOS which is a disease of hyperinsulinemia associated with infertility.

c) Reversing of DMT2 using a Low-Calorie diet for 3-4 months; losing 15kg or more leads to remission of DMT2 as evidenced by stopping of medications and HbA1c less than 6.5.

Reversing the irreversible: Type-2 Diabetes and You: Prof Roy Taylor (Manchester University) (43) "This study shows that half of the people with Type-2 Diabetes of duration less than 6 years can reverse their condition and remain "in remission" after 1 year. This is made possible by using a Very Low-Calorie Diet which leads to weight loss generally and leads to the recovery of the liver and pancreatic fat and normal HBA1c without the use of medications.

According to the Twin Cycle Hypothesis, long term intake of more calories leads to the accumulation of liver fat and hyperinsulinemia. Fatty liver leads to Very Low-Density Lipoprotein (VLDL) accumulation into all tissues including the pancreas which impairs Insulin secretion leading to Post Prandial Hyperglycemia and finally clinical Diabetes.

Low carbohydrate diets (ketogenic) have been used for the treatment of various diseases with strong evidence in:
1. Diabetes, weight reduction (obesity), epilepsy, hypertension, and reduction of cardiovascular risk parameters.
2. Emerging evidence in the treatment of Cancer, Polycystic Ovarian Syndrome (PCOS), neurological diseases e.g. Alzheimer's and Parkinson's diseases, and acne.

Beyond weight loss: A review therapeutic uses of very low carbohydrate ketogenic diet: A. Paolli (44) "This article explains ketosis and the therapeutic uses of ketogenic diets and gives:
a. Strong evidence in weight loss, cardiovascular disease, type-2 diabetes, epilepsy
b. Emerging evidence in acne, polycystic ovarian syndrome (PCOS), neurological disease e.g. headache, neuro-trauma, Alzheimer's disease and Parkinson's disease, sleep disorders, brain cancer, autism and multiple sclerosis, amyotrophic lateral sclerosis.

Other emerging applications of LCHF diets are in chronic pain syndrome, oxygen toxicity seizures, sports medicine, inflammation (arthritis) and migraine.

Emerging applications of the ketogenic diet: Dominic D'Agostino: A leading expert and researcher in ketogenic diets: (45). The clinical applications of ketogenic diets are due to its:
a) Anticonvulsant and neuroprotective effect.
b) Effect on glucose control, cancer metabolism, age-related inflammatory disorders
c) Improvement in Metabolic Biomarkers: Therefore ketogenic diets (nutritional ketosis) are used in the treatment/improvement of Metabolic Biomarkers.

In 1921 in Mayo Clinic, Ketogenic Diet (KD) was used clinically for seizures and to date, no antiepileptic drug is as effective as a ketogenic diet for all intractable seizure types.

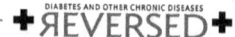
During the ketogenic diet, Carnitine deficiency can occur and its supplementation is recommended. Other deficiencies that can occur are Magnesium, Calcium, Sodium, and Potassium. Potassium deficiency can be corrected by Potassium citrate or vegetables.

Other supplements are Taurine and MCT oils.

There are many commercial types of exogenous ketones and also tools for assessing nutritional ketosis.

The Glucose/Ketone Index (GKI) is the ratio of blood glucose: Ketones and it is very valuable in the treatment of cancer and seizures. Its value should be maintained between 1 and 4 and this can be achieved by the ketogenic diet, modified Atkins diet, intermittent fasting, and exogenous ketones.

To validate the state of ketosis it is good to do the following biomarkers Cortisol, Insulin levels, and HbA1c.

The future direction for cancer therapy includes:
- Maintaining GKI of 1 to 4 by lowering insulin levels using ketogenic therapies
- Hyperbaric oxygen,
- IV vitamin C and
- Press and Pause Effect to eliminate the current use of Radiotherapy and Chemotherapy.

There is a lot of research interest on the Central Nervous System (CNS), toxic seizures, Alzheimer's disease, Angelman's Syndrome, anxiety behavior, stress, exercise performance, metabolomics, etc., cancer, wound healing, inflammation, longevity and disease prevention.

KEY TAKEAWAYS:

- *Low-Carb High-Fat (LCHF) diets are not new*
- *LCHF diet is the preferred diet for metabolic syndrome and type-2 diabetes.*

CHAPTER SEVEN

THE ROAD TO DIABETES REVERSAL

In 2016 I was on metformin, glibenclamide, pioglitazone and Conventional DMT2 diet. I used to have very severe backache, poor sight, numbness of feet and general body weakness. My sugars were erratic, sometimes my fasting blood sugars (FBS) was 14mmol/dl. I was following the path for DMT2 complications. DMT2 damages big and small blood vessels (micro vascular and macro vascular) leading to complications, which lead to progressive hypertension, eye damage (retinopathy), and cataracts causing poor vision, heart attacks (coronary heart diseases), progressive kidney damage (nephropathy), nerve damage (neuropathy), diabetic foot, leg amputations, Gastropathy leading to vomiting and diarrhea, urine retention and incontinence, erectile dysfunction etc. Maintaining normal blood sugars (glycaemia) is said to slow the progression of these complications.

I was following the diet as advised by the Nutritionist who was following the Kenya Diabetes Association Nutrition Guidelines. I made the necessary lifestyle changes including regular exercises, sleep, no smoking/drinking though I was still a bit obese with a BMI of 28. I was determined to get a solution to my DMT2 and became more interested in the history of the LCHF diet.

DR William Banting (1796-1867) started a low carbohydrate diet in 1867 at his doctor's behest after struggling with obesity. The diet Banting advocated was a low carbohydrate emphasizing meats, vegetables, and fruits; avoiding sugar and starch.

The South African Prof Tim Noakes popularized the *"The Banting Diet"* in South Africa after the release of his book, *"The Real Meal Revolution" (46)* The Book debunks the low fat "Lie" and shows the way back to restored health through eating what human beings are supposed to eat: a low-carb high-fat diet. This revolutionized the Banting Diet in South Africa.

In this diet, general foods allowed are avocado, low carbohydrate fruit, any dairy product (cream, butter), leafy green vegetables, and eggs, meat with fat, and fish and nuts. General foods to avoid are high carbohydrate vegetables and fruits, any processed foods, anything with added sugar, bread, oats, and pasta. Coconut oil and olive oil (for low heat cooking) are recommended.

The percentage of calories from macronutrients in low carb high-fat diets is 70% fat: 20% protein: 10% carbohydrate in Classical Ketogenic diet (CKD). The percentages vary in Modified (MCT) Ketogenic diet, Modified Atkins diet (MAD) and in Low Glycemic Index Therapy (LGIT).

The ketogenic diet (KD) has been used to treat children with epilepsy who are resistant to antiepileptic drugs since the 1920's.

LCHF diets are not universally standardized; a qualified Nutritionist/Dietician should be able to formulate the diet depending on locally available foodstuffs.

Some of the recommended low GI foodstuffs are not locally available or affordable e.g. Broccoli, cauliflower, asparagus, olive oil. Most Kenyan traditional foodstuffs have high to moderate GI e.g. Maize, peas, sorghum, beans, wheat products, and sweet potatoes.

I started intermittent fasting in November 2017. Initially, I was doing 18:6 i.e. fasting for 18 hours and eating between 2 PM and 8 PM.

In February 2018, I started my LCHF diet journey together with 30minutes of daily exercises and Intermittent Fasting (IF). I stopped consuming high GI foods e.g. maize, rice, wheat products, cassava, sweet potatoes, and Irish potatoes. I was eating a fistful (a serving spoon) amount of legumes per day i.e. peas/beans all types of meat (Serving spoon), a lot of vegetables (cooked/steamed/raw) 7-10 cups per day i.e. Sukuma wiki (kales), amaranth leaves (terere), managu, spinach, cabbage (fermented or steamed), carrots (few), tomatoes, okra, occasionally cauliflower, broccoli, zucchini, cucumbers, sugarless yogurt, and sugarless tea with ginger.

Initially, it was not easy. The craving for carbohydrates was overwhelming. I would get headaches, abdominal discomfort, daytime sleepiness, and insomnia.

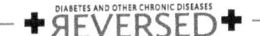
I was monitoring my blood sugars twice daily. After a few days on the LCHF diet and medications, my Random Blood Sugars (RBS) were going below 5mmol/dl, so I stopped taking pioglitazone, and the severe backache disappeared. Less than a month later I had to stop glibenclamide and metformin, my sugars were going below 5mmol/dl. By this point, I had lost weight and my BMI was down to 25. The feet numbness (peripheral neuropathy) was decreasing, my mood and sleep pattern had greatly improved, the brain fog disappeared; I was strong and energetic the way I used to feel twenty years prior. My vision improved, in less than four months my HbA1c dropped from 9.8 to 5.5. YES, I HAD REVERSED DIABETES!

KEY TAKEAWAYS:

- *Exercise, Intermittent Fasting and LCHF diet are the three main factors in reversal of diabetes type-2.*

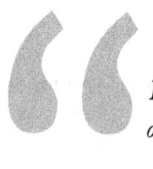

Initially, it was not easy. The craving for carbohydrates was overwhelming. I would get headaches, abdominal discomfort, daytime sleepiness, and insomnia.

CHAPTER EIGHT

THE LOW CARBOHYDRATE HIGH FAT KETOGENIC DIET CLINIC

I was working in a Rural Private Hospital and could see the sufferings of diabetic patients; frequent leg amputations, Diabetic Ketoacidosis (DKA) and other complications of DM and noticed that the number of diabetic patients was increasing.

I came across the work of English General Practitioner **DR David Unwin: Glycemic index: Helping patients in primary care: (47).** "DR Unwin gives the history of his frustrating work as a Practitioner in England for 25 years, managing diabetic patients with poor outcomes until he discovered the low carb diet group which was reversing diabetes and obesity and started applying it in the management of his diabetic patients. He read about the Glycemic Index (GI) and realized that the glycemic index for brown bread is higher than sugar.

Food Item	Glycaemic index	Serve size g	How does each food affect blood glucose compared with one 4g teaspoon of table sugar?
Basmati rice	69	150	10.1
Potato, white, boiled	96	150	9.1
French Fries baked	64	150	7.5
Spaghetti White boiled	39	180	6.6
Sweet corn boiled	60	80	4.0
Frozen peas, boiled	51	80	1.3
Banana	62	120	5.7
Apple	39	120	2.3
Wholemeal Small slice	74	30	3.0
Broccoli	15	80	0.2
Eggs	0	60	0

Other foods in the very low glycaemic range would be chicken, oily fish, almonds, mushrooms, cheese

Diabetes Type-2 is mainly about carbohydrate intake. He made an easy to understand GI of various foods in terms of spoons of sugar e.g. Basmati rice' GI is 69, a 150gm serving is equivalent to taking 10 spoonfuls of sugar. A banana with a GI of 62 is equivalent to 5.7 spoons of sugar. This scale made it easy for patients to understand the total sugar equivalence they were taking per meal and therefore enabled them to make the expected behavioral change. It is also important to agree with the patient on shared goals.

He had been treating Diabetic patients with conventional diet and medication for years with disappointing results. When Unwin started advising his patients to turn from conventional dietary guidelines to the LCHF (Ketogenic) diet, the results were astonishing. Most of his patients had their previously prescribed diabetic medications even Insulin injections withdrawn.

The case studies of 125 Consented patients helped by low carbohydrate diet in a primary care setting over an average of 15 months shows: a drop in HBA1c, gradual withdrawal of glycemic medications, weight loss, improved lipid profiles (decrease in total cholesterol, HDL, Cholesterol ratio, Triglyceride), blood pressure and liver function tests.

During our regular diabetic Outpatient Clinic we would teach the Conventional diabetic nutrition and lifestyle change, however I questioned; if DMT2 can be reversed and I had proven that fact, why should I withhold this valuable information from our patients? I invited some diabetic patients who had previously been treated in our health facility with severe diabetes to our Diabetic Clinic. I explained to them that although diabetes is said to be a chronic progressive disease, it can be reversed by a LCHF diet leading to the withdrawal of all diabetic medications. I took them through the local Low and High GI foods. One week later, one of the patients rang me enquiring whether to stop one of his diabetic (OHA) medications since his blood sugars were going down. I was not yet aware that he had heeded my advice to consider the LCHF diet. Within a month, all his diabetic medications were withdrawn and he was maintaining normal blood sugars by applying the LCHF diet. Other patients followed suit and in February 2018 our LCHF diet Outpatient Clinic was born.

The reorganized Outpatient Diabetic Clinic was following a Standard Patient Care Protocol which included:

a) Taking patient demographic details e.g. Name, weight, height, age, measuring blood pressure BP, heart rate, fasting blood sugar FBS, HbA1c

b) Etiology, signs and symptoms, diagnosis, types of diabetes, complications, conventional management of DM

c) Reversing DM by combining exercises, Intermittent Fasting (IF) and LCHF diet therapy. Other lifestyle changes e.g. stop smoking; minimize/stop alcohol consumption, stress management, sleep, eye, and foot care, screening for depression and managing stigmatization.

d) LCHF diet using locally available and affordable foodstuffs and demonstrations of the LCHF diet.

e) Personal experiences/testimonies from patients who have been on LCHF diets.

f) Personal One on One Doctor Patient Consultation.

Initially, the Outpatients were signing a Consent form and implementing the LCHF diet therapy at home and reporting any adverse effects to the hospital and getting any form of advice through mobile phones and subsequent clinic visits.

To ensure compliance with the diet, monitoring, safety, and treatment of any initial side effects we introduced Inpatient LCHF Therapy, which was compulsory for patients on injectable Insulin. Monitoring of blood sugars and ketones, and gradual withdrawal of diabetic medications was possible. The hospital personnel involved in the implementation of LCHF diet therapy included a multi-disciplinary team of a Registered Nutritionist/Dietician, Nurses, Pharmacy and Laboratory practitioners, a Chef and a Medical Doctor.

In 2018 I read widely on LCHF diet and its applications; I got most of the academic/clinical materials from Online books, Lectures, Scientific Journals and International Conferences e.g. Low Carbohydrate Down Under LC USA, the IHMC, Keto Salt Lake, Low Carb Denver, Virta Health, Diet Doctor, Low Carb Breckenridge, Ketocon Austin 2018, Ketofest 2018, Low Carb Houston, South African conference etc.

This background exposed me to leading Low Carb academicians e.g. DR Jason Fung, Prof Roy Taylor, DR Eric Westman, Dominic D"Agostino, DR Eric Kossof, DR Bret Scher, Nina Teicholz, DR Peter Attia, DR Zoe Hercombie, Prof Andrew Mente, DR David Diamond, DR Paul Mason, DR Dawn Lemanne, Prof Jeff Volek, Prof Tim Noakes, Ivor Cummins, DR Aseem Malhotra, DR Richard Bernstein, DR David Unwin and many others.

In 2018 and 2019 I undertook various online courses on the LCHF diet and its applications hosted by South African Prof Tim Noakes' NUTRITION NETWORK training in LCHF/Ketogenic Nutrition and Treatment in Clinical practice.

KEY TAKEAWAYS:

- *Glycaemic Index (GI) of carbohydrates is easier to understand in terms of spoons of sugar.*
- *The role of the dietician/ nutritionist in implementation of the LCHF diet is stressed*
- *The LCHF program at the hospital has proven to be more effective than any existing conventional interventions*
- *Monitoring, safety, and treatment of any initial side effects is vital*
- *Follow a Standard Patient Care Protocol.*

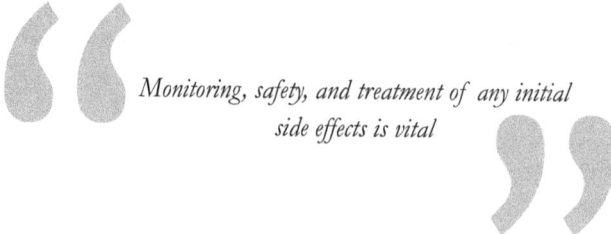

Monitoring, safety, and treatment of any initial side effects is vital

CHAPTER NINE

OBSERVATIONAL STUDY OF PATIENTS TREATED WITH LCHF DIET IN MULATYA MEMORIAL HOSPITAL, MAKUENI COUNTY, KENYA

Period of study February 2018 to July 2019 (analysis ongoing)

Total number of patients = 64

Diabetes Mellitus = 55

DMT1 = 1

DMT2 = 54

DMT2 + Hypertension = 43

DMT2 + Arthritis = 9

DMT2 + Gastropathy = 9

DMT2 + Retinopathy = 5

DMT2 + CVA = 3

DMT2 + Cardiomyopathy = 1

DMT2 + Pulmonary arterial hypertension = 1

DMT2 + Adult Epilepsy = 1

DMT2 + Parkinsonism = 1

Severe Hypertension without DM = 3

Severe arthritis without DM = 2

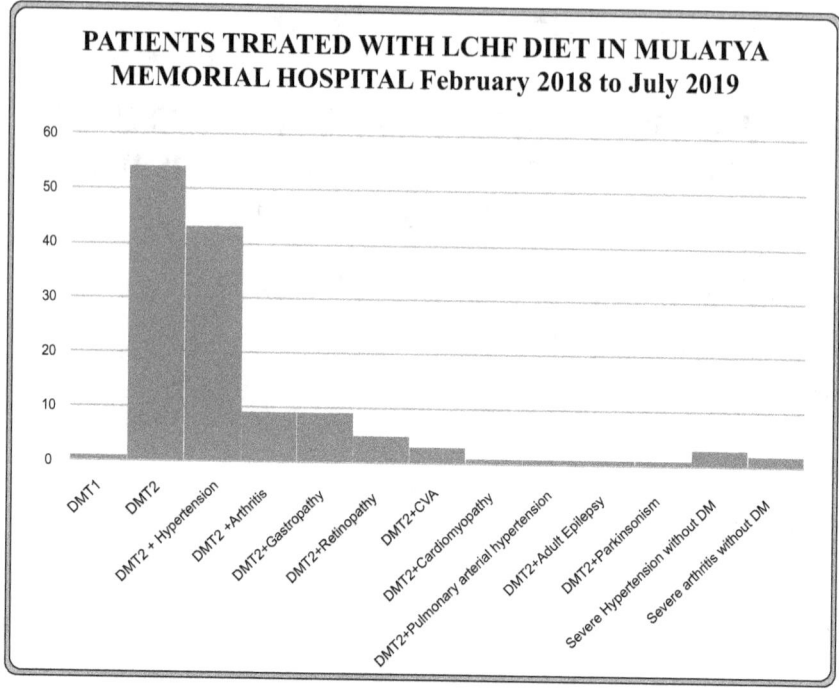

PATIENTS TREATED WITH LCHF DIET IN MULATYA MEMORIAL HOSPITAL February 2018 to July 2019

Most of the patients were DMT2 with associated diabetes complications and comorbidities. On admission, they were on oral hypoglycemic agents mainly metformin and glibenclamide or Mixtard Insulin and anti-hypertensive medications. After a maximum of 10-days Inpatient stay most of the oral hypoglycemic agents and insulin injections had been withdrawn. Some patients were discharged on Metformin; withdrawal of antihypertensive medications was achieved after 3-6 months Outpatient Clinic follow-up.

KEY TAKEAWAYS:

- *The observational study shows that LCHF is effective in the treatment of diabetes type-1, type-2, nephropathy and retinopathy, hypertension, severe arthritis, adult epilepsy and alzheimer's disease*
- *Besides the observational study, randomized controlled trials (RCT) are necessary*

CHAPTER TEN

MANAGEMENT OF TYPE-2 DIABETES (DMT2) WITH LCHF DIET

CASE STUDY 1

61-year old Male
Diagnosis:
- DMT2,
- Hypertension,
- Diabetic foot,
- Severe Rheumatoid arthritis,
- Obesity

July 2017

The patient presents with a history of severe joint pains, painful swellings and pus discharging wounds on the left foot. He has not been able to wear shoes for some months. General weakness, he takes some tablets for blood pressure on and off. On admission his B/P was high, he was febrile with what was thought to be cellulitis left foot. On examination, diagnosis made: hypertension, severe infected left foot and severe rheumatoid arthritis evidenced by tender deformed leg and elbow swellings (tophi) and characteristically deformed fingers. I suspected left diabetic foot since he was obese (weight 110Kgs) and requested for Random blood Sugar (RBS). He was arrogant; he knew he was not diabetic but after further persuasion, he agreed to the RBS which turned to be 29.5mmol/dl.

Diagnosis summary: DMT2 with left diabetic foot, hypertension, obesity, and severe Rheumatoid arthritis.

Management included soluble insulin, ceftriaxone injections, low dose aspirin, atorvastatin, Inj Metronidazole infusion, anti-hypertensive medications (amlodipine and losartan/HCTZ. He was discharged after 2 months for follow up in our outpatient diabetic clinic on mixtard insulin, low dose aspirin, amlodipine, losartan/hctz, and analgesics.

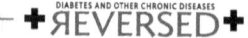
In February 2018, the patient was introduced to the LCHF diet under inpatient care and was later followed up in the weekly outpatient clinic. Within the first month, insulin injections were discontinued; within 6 months he had achieved glycemic control: normal sugars and HbA1c 5.5 from 10.2.

Low dose aspirin, atorvastatin, and oral hypoglycemic agents were withdrawn.

After 8 months of LCHF diet and gradual withdrawal of amlodipine and losartan/hctz, all antihypertensive medications had been withdrawn. His once severe rheumatoid arthritis improved considerably; he could walk without aid, the diabetic foot had healed and he could wear shoes. The patient had lost weight from an initial 110kg to 72kg and he had a normal BMI. A year later, he is pain-free and not on any medications. His B/P and HbA1c normalized; he regularly attends the clinic to encourage other patients on the effectiveness of the LCHF diet.

Discussion:

Reversibility of Type 2 Diabetes is currently possible by:
1. Bariatric surgery (BS).
2. Very low calorie (VLC) diets.
3. LCHF diets.

BS is expensive and sometimes irreversible and has long term complications. Very low calorie diet gives rapid improvement but has a high rebound in HbA1c and weight.

LCHF diet is as effective as BS, is safe, highly sustainable and leads to reduction in HbA1c, weight, glycemic medication reduction/discontinuation and inflammation reduction.

This case study is one of the many examples of successful reversal of DMT2 and its associated complications and comorbidities using a LCHF diet Therapy. Recent clinical studies have demonstrated that medically supervised individualized carbohydrate restriction can reverse DMT2 while eliminating glycemic control medications (OHA) gradually in days or months

Literature Review: the evidence of low carbohydrate nutrition for diabetics:
DR Amy Mackenzie (48) "Research on carbohydrate restriction for Insulin Resistance shows that low carbs were being used for control of diabetes in the pre-insulin era.

1. 2005 study: carbohydrate restriction works promptly leading to a fall in blood glucose, HbA1c, Insulin sensitivity "prior" to significant weight loss, medications reduced or eliminated, plasma triglycerides and cholesterol decreased and hunger reduced.

2. Long term (56weeks) effects of ketogenic diet among patients with obesity and diabetes: Fast improvement in glucose, weight loss, triglycerides, decreased LDL and HDL increase.

3. Longer-term effects (2 years) of a low carb diet compared with the Mediterranean and low-fat diets; weight loss at 2 years was greatest with low carb and Mediterranean (MED). HBA1c was only significant in the low-carb group. There was no calorie restriction in the low-calorie group.
   There is a greater reduction in HbA1c and diabetic medications with LCHF ketogenic diet versus a low glycemic index diet in patients with obesity and type-2 diabetes.

4. A very low carbohydrate diet achieves a greater reduction in HbA1c and medications at 3 months compared to a moderate carbohydrate diet.

5. A very low carbohydrate diet results in greater weight and HbA1c reduction at 6 and 12 months compared to a moderate carbohydrate diet.

6. Lower carbohydrate diet results in lower Triglycerides (TG), more medication reduction and lower HbA1c and glucose variability following 2 years compared to high carb/low fat/low GI diet.

7. Low fat diet (LFD) v/s Low Carb Ketogenic Diet (LCKD) for Atherogenic dyslipidemia and overweight/obesity: LCKD has more favorable impact on Metabolic Syndrome i.e. decreased body mass, abdominal fat, triglycerides, TG/LDL, Apo A, Apo B, small LDL, Glucose insulin, HOMA-IR, leptein, total saturated fatty acids (SFA), increased HDL.

8. A ketogenic diet has significant anti-inflammatory effects VS LFD: Seven out of 14 inflammatory markers significantly reduced.

Summary:

1. Insulin sensitivity and blood glucose rapidly improve with VLCKD
2. Sustained improvement in glucose, weight, and lipids at 1 and 2 years is possible with a low carbohydrate diet (LCD)
3. LCD can be better than low fat, Mediterranean, moderate carb and low glycemic index diets.
4. Calorie unrestricted lower (40% CHO intake) carbohydrate diets are a reasonable option for patients.
5. LCD reduces glucose variability over 2 years.
6. Very Low Carbohydrate Ketogenic Diets (VLCKD) improves markers of Metabolic Syndrome, reduces circulating saturated fatty acids and inflammation.

Eating patterns and diabetes:

More studies have been done on low carb than on DASH, Mediterranean and plant-based diets.

Studies on VIRTA Health research findings: (Indiana Reversal Study)
Results:

1. 60% of 1-year completers reversed diabetes; had sugar improvement HbA1c reduction 70% below 6.5.
2. Medication reduction: 60% of insulin users reduced or eliminated.
3. Weight loss: 12% average weight loss (30lbs)
4. CVD risk factor improvement:

> (12% improvement in 10year ASCVD risk score. 22 out of 26 risk factors improved)
> Patient retention was very high, at 83% at 1 year and 74% at 2 years.
> Most of the patients achieved and maintained nutritional ketosis as evidenced by blood levels of BHB, HbA1c improved rapidly and sustained at 2 years. Carbohydrate restriction improves HbA1c regardless of the starting level of glycemic control.
> LDL particle size moves from small to large.
> *Compared to statins: If LDL goes up after LCKD, do you consider a statin? No, because the LDL particle size moves from small which are Atherogenic to large.*
> Markers of NAFL disease improve significantly following Low Carb (LC) Nutrition.

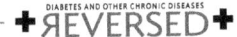
Substantive sleep quality improves after 1-year treatment with carb restriction.

Benefits of ketogenic diet for management of Type-2 diabetes: A review: Sami T Azar et al (49) "Ketogenic diet has several benefits on the management of type-2 diabetes which include reduction of HbA1c level, weight loss and improvement of lipid profiles; cardiac benefits, reversibility of neuropathy and even possible effect on reversing diabetic nephropathy and retinopathy".

Treatment of Diabetes and diabetic complications with a ketogenic diet Charles V. Mobbs et al: Review Article: (50), "Accumulating evidence suggests that Low Carb High Fat Diets (LCHF) are safe and effective to reduce glycemia in diabetic patients in humans and remarkably reduce blood glucose in Type-1 and 2 diabetes and reverse diabetic neuropathy in animal models.

Dietary interventions that include therapeutic levels of carbohydrate reduction can be used by Clinicians to achieve this goal, however many Clinicians have not been trained in how to administer these therapies. An inpatient setting is advisable.

A clinician's guide to low carbohydrate diets for the remission of Type-2 Diabetes: Towards a Standard care protocol: Mark Cucurella et al (51). This article outlines a seven-stage protocol for clinical practice guidelines and standard of care for doing carbohydrate reduction as an intervention for DMT2 and related conditions in an inpatient setting.

The standard of care protocol should consist of
 a) Patient selection
 b) Pre-diet evaluation and counseling
 c) Patient education
 d) Initiating of dietary intervention
 e) Managing medication changes
 f) Addressing any side effects and
 g) Follow up
 A Registered Food Service Dietician/Nutritionist is very essential in this protocol.

Currently, there are four methods to place DMT2 into remission: Bariatric Surgery, extended fasting, a very low-calorie diet using meal replacement formula **(48)** and LCHF diets.

The inpatient care setting for the implementation of the LCHF diets allows for a carefully controlled environment in which to change the diet, measure response and titrate medications appropriately. A new medication regimen can be safely established before discharge and Outpatient follow up.

The diabetic care protocol for Inpatient LCHF therapy was followed in our case study for reversal of DMT2 and associated complications like Diabetic foot, hypertension, and comorbidities (rheumatoid arthritis and obesity). Remission of DMT2 with LCHF diet therapy is indicated by the disappearance of signs and symptoms and measurement of HbA1c of 6.5mmol/dl with or without the use of Insulin sensitizing agents like metformin. Remission can be defined as two measurements below this threshold at two months apart again without the use of metformin.

Although the benefits of carbohydrate restriction for DMT2 patients are recognized, concerns are raised whether patients can adhere to this diet indefinitely because, in Conventional Nutrition, it is said that carbohydrates are an essential macronutrient. However, it is known that *dietary carbohydrate is not an essential nutrient: Institute of medicine US: National Press (52).*

a) Dietary carbohydrate is not an essential nutrient. An essential nutrient is one required for normal body function that CANNOT be synthesized by the body. Categories of essential nutrients include vitamins, dietary minerals, essential fatty acids, and essential amino acids.

b) *Is dietary carbohydrate essential for human nutrition?* **DR Eric Westman: (53)** "The theoretical lowest dietary carbohydrate intake is zero, provided that adequate amounts of protein and fat are consumed. The minimal amount of exogenous and endogenous carbohydrate is dependent on the brain (100-140g/dl per day).

A well-formulated LCHF diet which includes a variety of vegetables presents no health risks from nutritional deficits and is usually sustainable if incorporated as a lifestyle change.

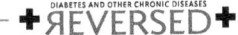

The American Diabetic Association (ADA) and European association for the study of diabetes (EAB) on 4th October 2018 ref (54) released a joint statement that included approval of low carbohydrate diet use in the management of DMT2 in adults. This came on the heels of Diabetes Australia releasing an updated position in August 2018 titled "Low carbohydrate eating for people with Diabetes".

The joint American and European position paper on the management of type-2 diabetes stated clearly *"There is no single ratio of carbohydrates, protein and fat intake that is optimal for every person with type-2 Diabetes".* The advantage of low carbohydrate diets in the management of type-2 diabetes in adults is that it is "inexpensive" and has no "side effects".

This statement stated that the recommendations are based on a 'systematic evaluation of literature since 2014' and have been followed by ADA consensus statement 2019. The role of a Registered Dietician or Nutritionist is stressed.

KEY TAKEAWAYS:

- *The low carbohydrate high fat diet reverses diabetes type-2 (DMT2), leading to discontinuation of medications.*
- *The theoretical lowest dietary carbohydrate intake is zero, provided that adequate amounts of protein and fat are consumed.*
- *Reversal of DMT2 leads to rapid improvement of HbA1c and is sustainable even after two years*
- *Many countries have officially approved the LCHF diet for reversal of DMT2 in adults.*

" *Dietary carbohydrate is not an essential nutrient. An essential nutrient is one required for normal body function that CANNOT be synthesized by the body.* "

CHAPTER ELEVEN

MANAGEMENT OF TYPE-1 DIABETES WITH LCHF DIET

CASE STUDY 2

This was a male patient 28 years old with mental sub-normality. An Electrical Technician diagnosed with DMT1 in 2013; on mixtard insulin 24/10IU, FBS 10 - 14. He was having occasional vomiting due to Diabetic Gastropathy; a complication of DMT1.

His B/P was normal and had an HbA1c of 10.5.

He was managed on the LCHF diet for 8 days as an inpatient and discharged on Mixtard insulin 10/5 IU.

Discussion:
Type-1 Diabetes (DMT1) is an Autoimmune Condition characterized by pancreatic *beta* cells destruction and absolute Insulin deficiency. The strongest predictor of diabetic complications is glycemic control. Achieving HbA1c of 7 or less is the primary management target.

Belinda S. Lennerz et al (55) study on the management of type-1 diabetes with a very low carbohydrate diet, was evaluating glycemic control among children and adults with type-1 Diabetes Mellitus who consume a Very Low Carbohydrate Diet (VLCD). They concluded that exceptional glycemic control of DMT1; with low rates of adverse events (i.e ketoacidosis or hypoglycemia) was rarely reported by a community of children and adults who consumed a VLCD.

4-10% of DMT1 patients die from hypoglycemia. The fear of hypoglycemia interferes with one's ability to achieve near-normal glucose control and it is the limiting factor in the glycemic control of DMT1.

A LCHF diet has been shown to reduce insulin requirements i.e. achieve normal glycemic control and lower hypoglycemic episodes.

Carbohydrate Restriction in Diabetes Management: DR Troy Stapleton: (56) a Radiologist diagnosed with Type-1 Diabetes Mellitus in 2012 and given standard dietary advice for 2 months then changed to low carb high-fat diet for 20 months. The Standard Dietary Advice (Food Pyramid) is 45-60gm carb with each meal times 3, 15-20gm carb snack times 2., total carb 240gm per day then adjust bolus insulin to carbohydrate intake e.g. Unit for 15gm of carbohydrates.

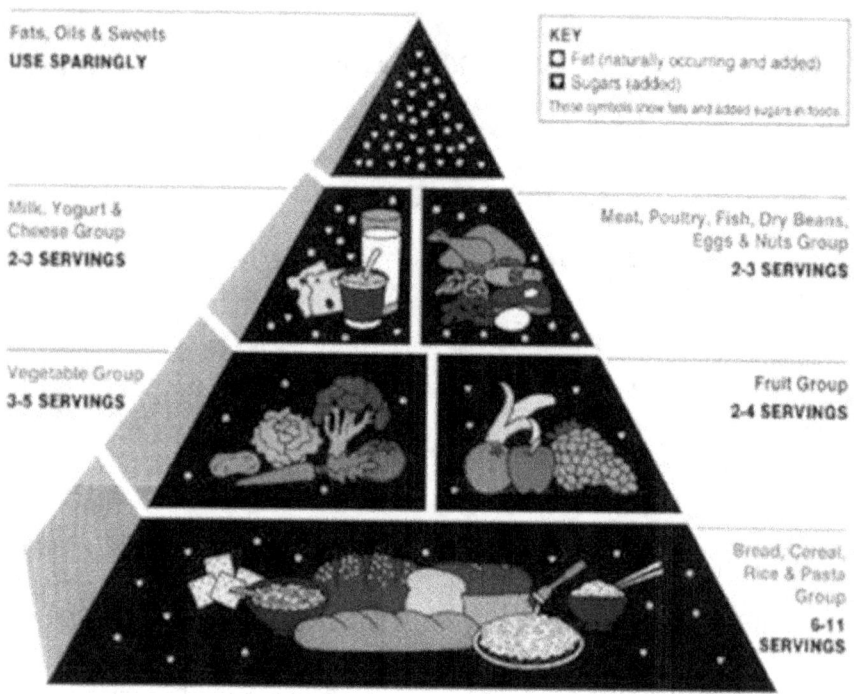

This is in line with Diabetes Australian Recommendation. To manage diabetes; your meals should be regular and evenly distributed throughout the day. It should be low in fat, particularly saturated fats, based on high-fiber carbohydrate foods e.g. whole grain bread, cereals, beans and lentils, fruits and vegetables.

After a lot of reading, he changed to Nutritional Dense foods, whole foods, VLCD/LCHF leading to Insulin dose of 10IU, mean glucose of 5.0, no spikes above 7.5, HbA1c of 5.2, and rarely had hypoglycemic attacks. After 20 months on the LCHF diet, he reduced to 10IU long-acting Insulin at night. HbA1c 5.2 (normal 4.3-6.0), rarely spiked, a BSL over 7.5mmol, rare hypoglycemic episodes, Triglycerides, HDL increased, B/P 124/76, weight 71kg, waist circumference 30", went back to surfing and cycling, improved mood and increased energy levels, with normal sustainable diet and no hunger.

He gives the story of:

1. **DR Keith Runyan:** DM LADA for 16 years: He is on LCHF diet, hypoglycemia ceased, HbA1c dropped to 5.0, Insulin dose dropped from 57 to 20 units per day, HDL-C increased to 65mg/dl, CRP decreased to 6.7mg/l, and he finished a triathlon without eating any food.

2. **Paul Buchanan** DMT1 at 44 years HbA1c at diagnosis was 13.4, went down to 5.1 within 4 months on LCHF diet; average less than 50gm carbs per day and 5-5.2% with rare hypoglycemic attacks, he participated in triathlons.

3. **Thanasis Bantios**: Has been on LCHF for 3 months. Previously when he was on a Conventional diet he was on high Insulin units and was getting hypoglycemic attacks. Now on the LCHF diet, he has a very reduced Insulin dose and is doing competitive wrestling without hypoglycemic attacks.

4. **DR Jones**: *I wish I had been told low carb was an option 20 years ago. Years of hypoglycemic spikes could have been avoided!*

   Diabetes management aims to normalize blood sugar and minimize hypoglycemia (decreasing HbA1c and glycemic variability). HbA1c reduction of 1% leads to a 14% decrease in risk of fatal and non-fatal myocardial infarction and a 31% decrease in microvascular endpoints e.g. kidney, eye.

The aims for diabetic treatment are to correct atherogenic dyslipidemia, reduce inflammation, blood pressure, encourage exercise, reduce weight/waist circumference, and minimize medications. (Insulin stimulates the sympathetic nervous system, reduces nitric oxide (NO) release from the endothelium and promotes smooth muscle proliferation).

A study in the LCHF diet in DMT1 long-term improvement and adherence: showed a reduction in HbA1c by 1.3%, mealtime insulin dose reduced from 23 to 13 units with stable basal insulin. Reduction in symptomatic hypoglycemia by 82%, HDL increased from 1.5 to 1.8. The total cholesterol/HDL ratio reduced from 3.9 to 3.5.

Another study in 2014 had similar results.

Summary:

In LCHF blood glucose lowers and stabilizes, reduces hypoglycemia, HDL rises, triglycerides reduce, visceral fat, weight, blood pressure, and LDL particles reduce.

Busted Myths on LCHF:

1. There is no evidence for adverse effects on kidney function. Reduction HbA1c and glycemic variability assist in preserving kidney function.
2. There is no evidence on the reduction of fiber in a LCHF diet; the shifting from flour and potatoes to fiber-rich leafy green vegetables.
3. There is no significant association between saturated fat and CVD.
4. Research supports VLCKD in humans.
   "The benefits of carbohydrate restriction for diabetes management are remarkable and documented, while the concerns about risk are conjectural and long term" Feinman R. et al.

Low Carbohydrate for Diabetes type-1 (DMT1): A systematic Review Jessica L Turton (57). "The standard treatment is dailyinjections of insulin and diet. Lowering HbA1c reduces the risk of micro and macrovascular complications in type-1 diabetes. Excessive use of insulin increases hypoglycemia risk and hyperinsulinemia which is associated with weight gain, Metabolic Syndrome, inflammation and Atherosclerosis, Alzheimer's disease and cancer.

The findings of the study were not conclusive but they suggested that Low Carb diet may assist in reducing or preventing hyperinsulinemia in type-1 diabetes by decreasing the absolute amount of Insulin required for tight glycemic control.

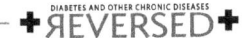
Management of type-1 diabetes with a ketogenic diet: Keith R. Runyan MD (58) "He outlines DMT1 after having been diagnosed with LADA. He was on exercise, Conventional diet, and insulin analogues but had frequent blood spikes and was on 57 units of insulin per day. Exercise led to deteriorating insulin control (Hypo and hyperglycemic episodes). Exogenous insulin does not mimic endogenous insulin.

DMT1 exogenous insulin results in hypoglycemia. During hyperinsulinemic hypoglycemia, liver glucose production remains suppressed thus not correcting hypoglycemia, this is called Defensive Glucose Counter Regulation.

Response to hypoglycemia varies; 4-10% of DMT1 patients die due to hypoglycemia. Fear of hypoglycemia limits glycemic control. DMT1 patients' inability to correct hypoglycemia results from Defensive Glucose Counter Regulation and hypoglycemic unawareness which is increased by recent hypoglycemic episodes, exercise, and sleep and alcohol ingestion. Severe hypoglycemia induces fatal cardiac arrhythmias.

In 2011 DR Runyan read "DR Bernstein's Diabetes Solution" and started LCHF in 2012. After the first 3 months on KD, he had decreased mean blood glucose, a 33% reduction in daily insulin dose, and a reduction in hypoglycemia frequency and severity. In KD ketones are used instead of glucose, preventing overt hypoglycemic reactions. Therefore Nutritional Ketosis prevents the adverse effect of hypoglycemia.

He was measuring blood ketones and occasionally taking supplements of BHB and MCT coconut oil during asymptomatic hypoglycemia. He has taken part in Professional Triathlon and weight lifting".

Carbohydrate intake and cardiometabolic risk factors in Type-1 Diabetes: Ail J Ahola et al (59) "Low carbohydrate diet (LCD) has gained interest among individuals with diabetes as a means to manage glycemia. The Finnish Diabetic Nephropathy Study examines adherence to the LCD and whether carbohydrate restriction is associated with cardiometabolic risk factors.

Higher carbohydrate-to-fat ratio was associated with higher blood glucose

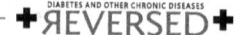
variability, higher blood pressure, and lower HDL cholesterol concentration and in men with lower waist-hip ratio.

Conclusion:

Reduced blood glucose variability, related to LCD could have clinical relevance to individuals with Diabetes type-1.

Conclusions

1. A well-formulated KD, daily exercise, frequent blood measurements, improve glycemic control and variability, symptoms of hypoglycemia, quality of life with lower insulin doses, lower risk of death and long term diabetic complications.
2. Glycemic variability is primarily due to exogenous insulin therapy.
3. Nutritional ketosis, exogenous ketones, and MCT fats may reduce hypoglycemic response by supplying the brain with ketones.
4. The numerous benefits of exercise outweigh the challenges of managing glycaemia with exercise in diabetes.
5. Beginning a KD for diabetics should be medically supervised.

Low insulin doses reduce the severity of hypoglycemic attacks and the onset of macro and micro vascular complications of DMT1.

"DR. Bernstein Diabetes Solution `"Book": (60) He was diagnosed with Diabetes at 12 years old. He developed diabetic complications at an early age: retinopathy, gastro paresis, cardiomyopathy, and nephropathy. He pioneered the blood sugar meter. He learned the relationship between carbohydrate intake and blood sugars and by adjusting his carbohydrate intake he could control his blood sugars throughout the day. He reversed his retinopathy, nephropathy, and depression by controlling his blood sugars. This book is not about food and exercise; a diabetic must take responsibility for his health.

From being diagnosed as a diabetic in 1946 to date, he is alive because of the measures he took. Bernstein started monitoring his blood sugars, he realized that dietary carbohydrates were contributing to his blood spikes and these could be reduced by restricting carbohydrates. The lower the carbohydrate intake the lower the insulin dose and the higher carb intake the higher the insulin dose.

Low dietary carbohydrate reduces blood sugar fluctuations. Bernstein recommends reducing carbohydrates as much as possible e.g. breakfast 6gm carbs, lunch 12gm carbs, dinner 12gm carbs, protein remains constant in the three meals. He recommends 30gm carbs daily: 6% not ADA's 250gm (50%) carb in a 2000calorie diet. For the prevention and treatment of hypoglycemia, he recommends taking a sugar cube.

DR Olivia Rimmington: Low Carb Nutrition in T1D (61): She was diagnosed with Type-1 Diabetes in 1996 having presented with the usual symptoms. She was given the Standard Conventional diabetic diet of 30gm carbs for breakfast, 45gm carbs for lunch and dinner leading to a rollercoaster of blood sugars. Like most of the children and adolescents with DMT1, she could not meet the recommended HbA1c of 7.1. Most of the DMT1 children and adolescents are overweight and Obese, and death rates are higher than the general population with a high rate of suicide.

High glucose (Hyperglycemia) is toxic and damages body cells. *So how can we improve diabetic outcomes?*

1. Improved blood sugar level (BSL) through intensive carb counting/Insulin management. But this also leads to an average weight gain of about 5Kg.
2. Strict glucose control of an average of 7% HbA1c delays long term diabetic complications and increases life expectancy.
3. But this increases the risk of hyperglycemia, severe hypoglycemia, and hypoglycemic hypo-awareness.

Why is intensive carb counting/insulin management difficult?

1. Mistakes in carb estimation which can be due to the net carb packaging etc.
2. Insulin absorption variability.
3. Insulin sensitivity varies with weight, hormones, exercise, duration of diabetes and weather.

4. Insulin resistance "Double Diabetes" especially in overweight/increased Insulin.

She discovered LCHF. She learned about DR Bernstein's Law of "Small Numbers"; eating small amounts of carbs and taking small amounts of insulin leads to predictable results and essentially normal blood sugar. Normal diabetic = Low carb = Normal BSLs.

How low should you go? Studies have shown that restricting carbs to less than 100gm per day can improve BSLs and reduce the risk of hypoglycemia. A very low carb/ keto diet (less than 30gm) per day, moderate protein and healthy fats to satiety leads to less insulin and more predictable stable BSLs.

The Bernstein Approach recommends 6gm carb for breakfast, 12gm for Lunch and Dinner and aims to keep protein portion for each meal constant. The low carb hypoglycemia management recommends using pure glucose, not fructose. I gm of pure glucose raises BSL by 0.3mmol/Litre. 3-4gm of pure glucose will raise BSL by 0.9-1.2mmols/Litre. Therefore this will bring normal BSL without rebound hyperglycemia.

Research supporting the Low-carb approach done in 2016-2018, Randomized Clinical Trial (RCT) Studies show that Low Carbs lead to average HbA1c of 5.67 and less hypoglycemic attacks with Bernstein's approach of less than 30gm Carbs per day.

LCHF diets lead to good glycemic control with very few hypos and hyper episodes, decreased HbA1c, the reversal of Retinopathy, weight loss and reduced insulin dose.

Summary:
1. With a LCHF diet, Insulin may decrease by 50%.
2. You cannot use fixed insulin doses.
3. Basal Insulin doses may also require adjustment.
4. Treat protein with Insulin NOT free e.g. 10gm Protein= 6gm Carb, therefore cover with Actrapid Insulin/duo wave bolus.

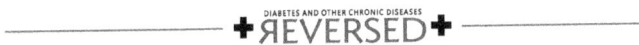

Continuous glucose monitoring is expensive, helpful but not essential. Frequent blood sugar testing (6 times a day ideally) pre and post meals is recommended because if you don't know your blood glucose it is harder to fix it and it will also enable detection of asymptomatic hypoglycemia.

Difference between nutritional Ketosis (NK) and DKA:
NK is a benign metabolic state, the body uses fatty acids from dietary fat or ketones made from fat instead of glucose as a primary energy source. This allows human metabolism flexibility to deal with famine/major shifts in dietary fuels. Ketone levels are usually 0.3-3mmol/Litre.

DKA is an unstable and dangerous condition due to Insulin deficiency or withheld insufficiency of exogenous Insulin. Ketones are usually more than 3mmols/Litre (up to 15-25), there are high BSLs and symptoms e.g. Nausea and vomiting, increased thirst, frequent urination, and abdominal pain.

Carbohydrate intolerance may accompany Nutritional Ketosis; the change in metabolic machinery can make it difficult to oscillate between low Carb and high Carb. This is likely related to peripheral insulin resistance (to prevent hypoglycemia).

Australia Diabetic Association acknowledges that Low Carb can be used in Type-1 Diabetes Mellitus (DMT1).

Final Thoughts:
1. *Current dietary guidelines are associated with poor outcomes for DMT1!*
2. *Low Carb offers DMT1 hope that there is another way to improve their glycemic control and avoid premature death.*
3. *All type-1 Diabetics deserve to know that Low Carb is an option!*

Sam M Scott: Carbohydrate restriction in type-1 diabetes: A realistic therapy for improved glycemic control and athletes performance: (62). The history of carbohydrate and calorie restriction dates back to the Pre-Insulin era. This was the only way of delaying death from ketoacidosis.

The 1960's recommendations shifted to a reduction of fat intake (less than 35% of energy) and increased carbohydrate intake to roughly 50 to 55% of total energy intake. The concept of matching insulin to carbohydrate intake, rather than food intake matched to estimated energy needs and insulin dosages, has become Standard Practice in DMT1 management.

The ADA Standard of Medical Care in Diabetes (2018) recommends 15 to 20% of total energy from protein, 20-35% of energy from dietary fat and 45-60% energy from carbohydrates; these macronutrient guidelines are similar in children and adolescents with DMT1. A low carbohydrate diet (LCD) 50-130gm of carbohydrate per day is more realistic.

For athletes, carbohydrate requirements should follow a sliding scale and be adjusted on the daily training day by day, meal per meal depending on daily training and competition schedule. Elite athletes have been found to perform well on a low carbohydrate diet.

LCDs in DMT1 can reduce glycemic variability, body weight and time spent in hypoglycemia. The potential benefits of low carbohydrate diets in people with DMT1 are:

1. Prevent and treat overweight and obesity in DMT1 due to decreased caloric intake and insulin dosage.
2. Prevent the treatment of hypoglycemia with more carbohydrate snacks. Chronic exogenous insulin use leads to increased Insulin Resistance an independent risk factor for microvascular (Neuropathy) and macrovascular (coronary and peripheral vascular disease) complications in DMT1.
3. LCD leads to a reduction in HbA1c. However, in patients taking Sodium-Glucose Co-Transporter (SGLT2) inhibitors, very low carbohydrate diets (VLCD) may lead to Euglycemic DKA. LCD may lead to increased LDL and this may be beneficial.
4. A well-formulated LCD does not lead to nutritional deficiencies.

Exercise significantly increases the risk of hyperglycemia and hypoglycemia in people with DMT1. Maintaining blood sugar levels within acceptable range before, during, and after exercise requires a balance between correct insulin doses, carbohydrate, and protein intake.

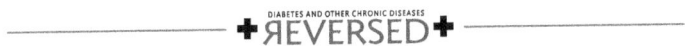
Carbohydrate restriction requires nutritional strategies for the endurance athlete with DMT1 e.g. twice a day training, fasted exercise, sleep low-train low.

Conclusion

Sensible LCDs consisting of less than 130 gm per day carbohydrates improve glycemic control and metabolic health in DMT1 leading to a reduced risk of hypo and hyperglycemia and reduced insulin requirements.

In our case study on DMT1, we managed to reduce insulin (Mixtard) dose from 24/10 to 10/5 IU. It is important to know whether a patient is DMT1 or DMT2, or Latent Autoimmune Diabetes of Adulthood (LADA) so as to predict the outcome of the LCHF diet therapy.

LADA is a form of diabetes type-1 that develops later in adulthood. It tends to develop more slowly than type-1 diabetes in childhood and sometimes appears similar to diabetes type-2 and can easily be mistaken for type-2 diabetes.

Paolo P et al (63) " LADA: Current status and new horizons: gives a detailed account of the epidemiology of LADA, genetic features, autoimmunity, the difference between LADA and DMT2, differences in clinical and genetic features between LADA and DMT1, complications and treatment.

Cameron F J et al (64) "Maturity onset diabetes of the young (MODY): discusses three case reports and a new perspective" outlines that MODY is a rare type of juvenile diabetes that presents with hyperglycemia in the absence of ketosis. Three cases who had pedigrees with diabetics in multiple generations presented in adolescence with evidence of insulin resistance; two were relatively overweight. All were readily controlled on diet alone.

Maturity onset diabetes of the youth (MODY): Health Topics (65) and Agarwal et al(66) "outlines clinical onset, genetic heterogeneity in MODY and treatment with diet /OHA and insulin.

Conclusion:

There is anecdotal evidence that MODY and LADA types of diabetes do benefit from the LCHF diet leading to deprescription of all oral hypoglycemic agents (OHA) and/or reduction in insulin doses while maintaining HbA1c of less than 6%.

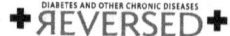

The following laboratory investigations should be done: C-peptide, Anti GAD or/and islet antigen 2 (IA2). Remember c-peptide levels are suppressed by insulin injections.

Anti-glutamine acid decarboxylase (Anti-GAD) is a marker of autoimmune antibodies.

KEY TAKEAWAYS:

- *A low carbohydrate high fat diet leads to the reduction of insulin dose, severity, and frequency of hypoglycemia (low blood sugar).*
- *Low insulin dose delays macro vascular (large) and micro vascular (small) vessel damage due to diabetes.*
- *A well-formulated LCD does not lead to nutritional deficiencies.*
- *Low Carb offers DMT1 hope that there is another way to improve their glycemic control and avoid premature death.*
- *Current dietary guidelines are associated with poor outcomes for DMT1!*
- *Maturity Onset Diabetes of Youth (MODY) and Latent Autoimmune Diabetes of Adulthood (LADA) types of diabetes do benefit from LCHF diet*

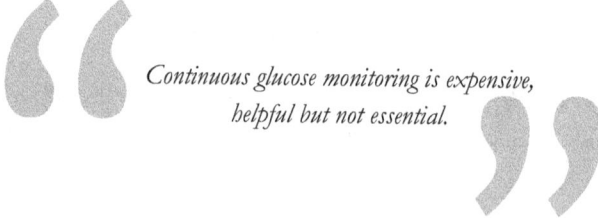

Continuous glucose monitoring is expensive, helpful but not essential.

CHAPTER TWELVE

MANAGEMENT OF HYPERTENSION WITH LCHF DIET

CASE STUDY 3

The patient was a 48-year-old male with DMT2 which was diagnosed 5-years prior. He was on metformin and Mixtard Insulin 30/20 IU. He was also a hypertensive on Nifedipine and Losartan/HCTZ.

He had had a skin-grafted left foot due to severe diabetic foot.

He was started on LCHF diet therapy, changed to soluble insulin. Complete but gradual withdrawal of soluble insulin and oral antihypertensives had been achieved by day 5.

He was discharged on the 10th day with normal B/P, RBS, and FBS with no medications.

Follow up after 6 months: normal B/P, and HbA1c 5.7 while on a LCHF diet.

This was the most remarkable and fastest response of Diabetes Type-2 and hypertension to the LCHF diet that we witnessed.

Discussion:
Hypertension is the most modifiable factor for Coronary Heart Disease (CHD). In our Observational Study, 43 out of 55 i.e.78% diabetic patients had associated hypertension. Treatment of hypertension includes lifestyle modifications e.g. weight loss, alcohol reduction, reduction of salt intake, adequate dietary Potassium, Calcium, and Magnesium, stop smoking, regular exercises and antihypertensive medications. The LCHF diet is associated with the improvement of risk factors associated with hypertension e.g. diabetes, obesity, and abnormal lipid profiles.

In our Observational Study, 3 patients had hypertension without Diabetes Mellitus. After patient admission, LCHF diet and Outpatient follow up, their antihypertensive medications were withdrawn gradually. The reduction in the severity of hypertension can be due to the effect of the LCHF diet on obesity but for the above patient, the drop in blood pressure and discontinuation of medications within five days could not have been due to weight loss.

Dr. David Unwin (67) in the Observational Study in Insulin Resistance Patients in Primary Care: shows that substitution of high carbohydrate diet with low carb diets for an average of 2 years enable:

1. Improvement in blood pressure to require adjustment or discontinuation of medications.
2. Reduction in body weight.
3. Improvement in lipid parameters.

Effective and a Novel Case Model for the Management of DMT2 at 1 year: Hallberg S. J et al (68) demonstrates that a novel metabolic and continuous remote care model can support adults with DMT2 to safely improve HbA1c, weight and other biomarkers while reducing diabetes medication use.

In a recent study on patients who have been on a LCHF diet, 10-year ASCVD risk decreased by 2%, B/P medications stopped in 12%, small LDL–P decreased by 20%, TG/HDL decreased by 29%, and large VLDL decreased by 30%.

KEY TAKEAWAYS:

- *Hypertension is the most modifiable factor for Coronary Heart Disease*
- *A low carbohydrate high fat diet improves blood pressure leading to adjustments or discontinuation of medications.*
- *The LCHF diet is associated with the improvement of risk factors associated with hypertension*

CHAPTER THIRTEEN

TREATMENT OF ADULT EPILEPSY AND LYMPHEDEMA WITH LCHF DIET

CASE STUDY 4

The patient was a 62-year-old female, with DMT2, Hypertension, Epilepsy, and Lymphedema.

The patient had been on treatment for hypertension and epilepsy for more than 5 years and had bilateral leg swelling (lymphedema) and DMT2 for a 1-year duration

She was on the following medications: (OHA) Metformin, Glibenclamide, Losartan, amlodipine, carbamazepine (Tegretol), Levetiracetam (Keppra).

She was admitted for 10 days for LCHF diet Therapy, metformin and glibenclamide were discontinued on discharge.

Outpatient follow-up: Carbamazepine was discontinued after 2 months, while Levetiracetam was discontinued after 4months.

Amlodipine was discontinued after 2 months, losartan after 6 months

After 9 months of outpatient follow-up on LCHF diet therapy with no medications, the patient maintained a normal B/P, HbA1c of 5.8 and no convulsions were experienced. Lymphedema had decreased significantly.

1. The management of DMT2 and hypertension using the LCHF diet has been discussed and this patient further confirms the efficacy of the diet.

2. **Lymphedema**: Lymphatic disorders do respond to a LCHF diet though the response can be gradual as it was in this patient.

Ketogenic Way of Eating for Lymph Disorders DR Eric Westman: An Obesity Medicine Specialist (69) "Studies on ketogenic diet and lymphedema have been going on. It is safe to lower carbs. The minimum dietary carbohydrate requirement is zero. The range of dietary carbohydrate is from 300gm a day (typical American diet) to less than 20gm per day (ketogenic diet). There are high and low glycemic index foods. The brain can utilize ketones instead of glucose.

The history of the low carb diet dates back to the Banting diet in 1893.

Ketogenic diets lead to weight and fat mass loss in patients affected by obesity. Metabolic Syndrome leads to cardiovascular disease, Type-2 diabetes, and atherogenic dyslipidemias.

Low-fat diets lower LDL-C but low carb ketogenic diets lower all metabolic syndrome parameters including a decrease in blood pressure, obesity, diabetes, weight and improvement in lipid profiles. HbA1c is much reduced by LCKD than by low GI diets; Insulin and hypoglycemic medications are reduced or eliminated gradually.

Summary:

a) Ketogenic diet leads to reduced hunger and a spontaneous reduction in calorie intake.

b) Ketogenic diet leads to improvement in obesity, Metabolic Syndrome, type-1 and type-2 Diabetes.

c) The ketogenic diet can be used in a clinical setting for many chronic diseases.

d) Preliminary research suggests that ketogenic diets may assist in treating lymphedema and lipedema.

Diet and Lifestyle for Lymphatic disorders: Leslyn Keith: (70) "She outlines her research in obesity and lymphedema, current and future research, Nutrition and Lymphatic Health, implementation of a ketogenic way of eating and resources.

In the ketogenic way of eating (LCHF), the fuel source changes from glucose to fat. The Adipose tissues store the preferred fuel source, and is a meaningful way of weight loss without muscle loss.

Benefits of the LCHF diet include treatment of epilepsy, cancer, (Warburg effect), hyperlipidemia, cardiovascular disease, type-2 diabetes, weight loss, neurological conditions (Alzheimer's disease), and lymphatic diseases.

The worldwide obesity epidemic coincides with the 1977 US Dietary Guidelines.

Weight loss using the ketogenic diet will significantly impact lymphedema and quality of life (QOL). Results from various Clinical Trials show that ketogenic diets affect all parameters of weight loss except body mass. Lymphedema exclusively affects women and there is disproportionate adipose distribution to the lower half of the body, hypersensitivity and pain and easy bruising. Lymphedema is widely believed to be resistant to diet and exercise but there are many studies showing that it responds to the ketogenic diet.

Ketogenic way of eating in patients with or without obesity leads to lymphatic health because of:

a) Reduction of adipose tissue in a lymph edematous limb; lymph is lipophilic, and there is lipolysis associated with acute inflammation and lipogenesis associated with chronic inflammation.

b) Improved metabolic health and blood panel changes.

c) Improved immune function leading to reduced inflammation, facilitation of wound healing, improvement of skin condition and fewer infections.

d) Decreased edema due to reduced inflammation and improved drainage.

The ketogenic diet can lead to a reduction of adipose tissue in the lymphedematous limb, post-mastectomy. There is a decrease in swelling of the limb, weight loss and lipid panel improvement, improved cognition, and pain.

In lymphedema without obesity, KD leads to reduced limb volume. Exercise can increase or decrease limb swelling depending on intensity.

3. **Adult epilepsy:** Since its introduction in 1921, the ketogenic diet has been used in children with difficult to control seizures. Many studies on the effect of ketogenic diets in the management of adult epilepsy have been done e.g. Mayo Clinic and John Hopkins in the USA. The results are similar to those in children, after three months, 47% had a 50% reduction in seizures just like in children

Ketogenic diets in adolescents and adults with epilepsy: Neil M. et al (71) "The ketogenic diet is an alternative treatment for patients with refractory epilepsy. Most studies report dietary response in children but there is limited data evaluating the efficacy of ketogenic diets in adults. This study concluded that the ketogenic diet can be safely used in adults and adolescent population with a response similar to those seen in children. Patients with symptomatic generalized epilepsy may be particularly good candidates for this type of dietary treatment.

Payne N E et al: The ketogenic related diets in adolescents and adults: A review: (72). The KD and its variants may lead to similar seizure stoppage and reduction in seizure frequency in adolescents and adults. It outlines the composition of ketogenic diets (KD) and its variants.

DIET	Ketogenic Ratio	% Carbs	% Protein	% Fat LCT	%Fat MCT
Classical KD	4:1	4	6	90	0
MCT Diet	3:1	19	10	11	60
Modified MCT	3:1	19	10	41	30
Modified Atkins Diet (MAD)	1:1	10	25	65	0
LGIT	0.6:1	10	30	60	0

1. Classical KD is effective in the reduction of seizure frequency and freedom in drug-resistant epilepsy in adolescents and adults like in children.

Most side effects were mild and readily managed: nausea/vomiting, constipation, abdominal cramps, increased cholesterol and serum lipids, and weight loss.

1. MAD side effects are similar to classical KD. It has nearly the same seizure reduction frequency and freedom.
2. Effectiveness of LGIT: appears to be like KD but tolerability is poor.

Conclusion

KD and its variants may be effective in almost half of adolescents and adults with drug-resistant epilepsy. Side effects are transient and most common reason for discontinuation of treatment is lack of effectiveness.

Ketogenic Diets for Epilepsy: A century of Progress: DR Eric Kossoff (73)
"Fasting and dietary manipulation for the treatment of Epilepsy is mentioned in Bible times in Mark 9:14-29.

In 1921 Mayo Clinic started High-Fat low-Carbohydrate to mimic fasting state for children with epilepsy. Anticonvulsant drugs developed in the 1940s and 1950s to today's third-generation anticonvulsants which gave patients an easier option for control of epilepsy but resulted in a decline in the use of the diet for treatment of epilepsy. In the early 1990s diet was used as a last result and perceived as "alternative Medicine. Charlie Foundation in 1993 boosted the use of the ketogenic diet. Since then many books have been written and research have been done. The argument was that there were few randomized control trials but the Cochrane study (2012) Review of all the literature concluded: These studies suggest that in children, *the ketogenic diet results in short to medium term benefits in seizure control, the effects of which are comparable to modern antiepileptic drugs"*.

Ketogenic diets today are used in Epilepsy Centers:

1. Used typically after two drugs have been tried.
2. As one of the 4 major mainstream treatments: Medication, electrical stimulation, Epilepsy surgery, and dietary intervention.
3. It is much easier today for families with an interest in low carb diets for health.

Traditional initiation of the ketogenic diet: Traditionally started in the hospital for 2 to 4 days; it starts with 24 hours fasting, Dieticians calculate ratios (fat, protein and carbohydrates, fluids), offer daily education of families, and foods are measured.

Maintenance: Children are seen every 3 to 6 months for lab examinations, Dietician and neurological evaluation to assess efficacy and safety. After 2 years if successful (3 months, if not) in children the ketogenic diet is slowly weaned back to previous foods.

How can we make the ketogenic diet more flexible?
   a) In how to start: no fasting, no admission but gradual introduction of the diet.
   b) Four different KD all with nearly similar results
      • Standard KD
      • Medium-chain triglyceride (MCT) diet.
      • Modified Atkins Diet (MAD).
      • Low Glycemic Index Treatment (LGIT).
   c) No reason for fluid or calorie restriction.
      All four diets are equally valid; each Center should choose the diet they want to apply but Standard KD is for less than 2 years, Modified KD (MAD) for patients who are more than 12 years old.
      80% of the Centers admit for the diet but 92% say it is optional, 28% fast at the start although 68% say it is optional. Fasting is not recommended in infants less than 2 years old.
   d) Supplementation: Multivitamins, calcium, selenium, and salt are optional. Is it possible to take ketogenic tablets instead of the diet e.g. ketogenic esters?

In adults, the seizure response to KD is the same as in children. Questions in adults are;
   • Improving compliance, lipid profile changes and safety of the KD in pregnancy; evidence so far shows that it is safe.
   • In the developing world check the minimum requirements to start a KD Center.

- Guidelines of setting a Dietary Epilepsy Intervention Centre are available in International League against Epilepsy (ILAE), Ketogenic diet articles *Epilepsia Vol. 56 issue 9.*
- Flexibility and supplements have made the diet safer and easier "Metabolic based treatments" are now an entire new Anticonvulsant Class.

More than 50% of the adult patients have seizure reduction on the classic ketogenic diet (KD) and 12-61% for the modified Atkins diet has been demonstrated.

The Role of Ketogenic Diets in Epilepsy and Status Epilepticus: Tanya (74)
"This is a very detailed Article which covers
1. Introduction of ketogenic diets
2. Efficacy and indications in adults
   - Management of chronic epilepsy
   - Management of Refractory Status Epilepticus; various clinical trials and outcomes using ketogenic diets
3. Guidelines for implementation and maintenance with ketogenic diets and Modified Atkins diet (MAD)
4. Adverse effects, compliance and appropriate management

Conclusion:
Ketogenic diets offer an increasingly needed adjunct to antiepileptic drugs in the management of chronic epilepsy and refractory status epilepticus in adults.

Our case study patient lost about 5Kg in 9 months and looked young and happy; she had stopped all medications but she is still on the LCHF diet.

KEY TAKEAWAYS:
- *Lymphedema/Lymphatic disorders do respond to a LCHF diet though the response can be gradual*

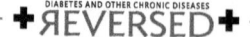

- *Adult drug-resistant epilepsy responds to Low carbohydrate high fat diet, leading to gradual withdrawal of medications.*
- *Various LCHF diet types are effective in Adult epilepsy*

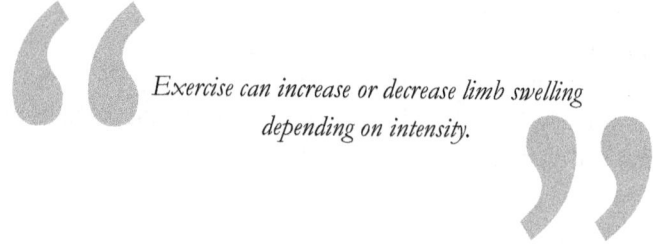

Exercise can increase or decrease limb swelling depending on intensity.

CHAPTER FOURTEEN

TREATMENT OF CARDIOMYOPATHY WITH LCHF DIET

CASE STUDY 5

The patient was a 55-year-old Male diagnosed with DMT2, two-weeks prior. He was a smoker and drinks alcohol. He was on Chlorpropamide (diabenese) and glibenclamide.

On examination, the patient had a puffy face, leg edema, B/P 129/99, had hepatomegaly and was very dyspnoeic. Chest X-ray indicated massive cardiomegaly. The echocardiogram done showed that he had Cardiomyopathy.

On admission, he was treated with Spironolactone, carvedilol, furosemide, and losartan.

Fasting Blood Sugar (RBS) was 12.6.

Day 1: patient was started on LCHF diet Therapy.

Day 2: patient had severe respiratory distress and he was put on oxygen, the above treatment, and vitamin B complex.

By Day 5: dyspnea was decreasing.

By day 10: the patient was discharged on Spironolactone, furosemide, carvedilol, and LCHF diet.

Follow up after one month: He had no leg edema and blood sugars had normalized.

Outpatient Clinic follow-up after 3 months: The patient was stable on furosemide, carvedilol and had dyspnea on exertion.

Discussion:
This patient had DMT2 and cardiomyopathy. Hypertrophic cardiomyopathy is often associated with hypertension, obesity, and DMT2.

There are several factors that cause diabetic cardiomyopathy such as autoimmune dysfunction, interstitial fibrosis, increased oxidative stress, mitochondrial dysfunction and myocardial stiffness due to persistent hyperglycemia with glycation of interstitial protein.

Very few studies have been reported on the use of the LCHF diet in cardiomyopathy. The patient in our observational study responded well to a LCHF diet.

Improvement of Cardiomyopathy after High-Fat diet in two siblings with Glycogen Storage Disease Type III: Alexandra Brambilla et al (75) "The two patients had Severe Progressive Cardiomyopathy which could not be maintained on high protein and *beta*-blockers. The high fat, medium protein, and low carbohydrate diet led to dramatic improvement in clinical conditions, biochemical and echocardiographic findings".

More studies are needed to ascertain the role of the LCHF diet in the treatment of congestive cardiac failure (CCF) and Cardiomyopathies.

Aubert G et al: 2016: The failing heart relies on ketone bodies as fuel (76). "Significant evidence indicates that the failing heart is energy-starved. During the development of heart failure, the capacity of the heart to utilize fatty acids the chief fuel diminishes.

In this study quantitative mitochondrial proteomics was used to identify energy metabolic derangements that occur during the development of cardiac hypertrophy and heart failure in well-defined mouse models. The results indicate that the hypertrophied and failing heart shifts to ketone bodies as a significant fuel source for oxidative ATP production.

Diabetic Gastro Paresis: Principles and Current Trends in Managements: Sathya Krishnasamy et al (77) "This is a very comprehensive review of Diabetic Gastro Paresis as a component of autonomic neuropathy resulting from long-standing poorly controlled type-1 and type-2 diabetes. It includes diagnosis, nutritional dietary management, lifestyle modifications, glycemic management, pharmacological and surgical management.

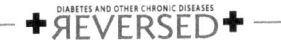
The Review points to the fact that *the cardiac muscle prefers free fatty acids (FFA) than glucose*: Nutritional Ketosis due to LCHF diet shifts myocardial fuel metabolism from fat/glucose oxidation to more energy-efficient fuel, ketone bodies and improves myocardial work and function to failing heart in CCF.

Ketogenic Diets in Endocrine Disorders: Current Perspectives: L. Gupta (78)
"Ketogenic diet (KD), a high fat, adequate-protein, and low carbohydrate diet leads to nutritional ketosis and is long known for antiepileptic effects; it has been used therapeutically to treat refractory epilepsy. This review attempts to summarize the evidence and clinical application of KD in diabetes, obesity, and other endocrine disorders. An Indian variant of the ketogenic diet has been provided. *The KD has beneficial effects on cardiac ischemic preconditioning,* improves oxygenation in patients with respiratory failure, improves glycemic control in diabetes, is associated with significant weight loss and has a beneficial impact on polycystic ovarian syndrome (PCOS).

Multivitamin supplements are recommended with KD. Recently ketones are being proposed as a super metabolic fuel, and the KD is currently regarded as an apt dietary therapy for "diabesity".

KEY TAKEAWAYS:

- *Cardiac muscle prefers free fatty acids to glucose*
- *The failing heart shifts to ketones produced by the LCHF diet for fuel.*
- *LCHF diet is cardioprotective*

"

During the development of heart failure, the capacity of the heart to utilize fatty acids the chief fuel diminishes.

"

CHAPTER FIFTEEN

TREATMENT OF PULMONARY ARTERIAL HYPERTENSION WITH LCHF DIET

CASE STUDY 6

The patient was a 65-year-old male; he was diagnosed with pulmonary arterial hypertension (PAH), DMT2, Benign Prostatic Hypertrophy (BPH), Lumbar Disk prolapse and Hypertension.

Medications were Clopidogrel, Irbesartan (Irovel) and was on follow up by a Cardiologist.

The patient developed sudden weakness, dyspnea while on a journey and was admitted into our Health facility. PAH medications were temporarily stopped except clopidogrel.

On admission, his B/P was 110/70, FBS 6.1 and was started on the LCHF diet for 10 days.

Within 10 days of admission, B/P, FBS, RBS were normal and there was a progressive decrease in dyspnea.

Outpatient Clinic follow-up up to 3 months: medications for pulmonary arterial hypertension were gradually withdrawn.

He was on a maintenance dose of clopidogrel and was able to walk a long distance i.e. his Six Minute Walk Distance (6MWD) had improved considerably.

Discussion:
Multiple studies have shown the inflammatory basis of pulmonary arterial hypertension. The release of adipokines causes a constant state of inflammation which could serve as a link between obesity and pulmonary arterial hypertension.

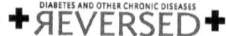

LCHF ketogenic diet can be tolerated, leading to weight loss, and be associated with clinical improvement in a patient with PAH on systematic prostacyclin therapy.

*Ketogenic Diet in Group 1 Pulmonary Hypertension Patient: J. Dyer (79)*Discussed is the improvement of a 48-year-old female patient with Pulmonary Arterial Hypertension (PAH) on ketogenic diet necessitating reduction of treprostinil dosage, reduced shortness of breath and improvement in 6-minute walk distance (6MWD). This could have been due to the weight loss and or anti-inflammatory effect of the ketogenic diet.

In our case study improvement could have been due to weight loss and the anti-inflammatory ketones (especially *beta*-hydroxybutyrate) produced by LCHF ketogenic diets but the duration was very short for the weight loss to have been a contributing factor.

KEY TAKEAWAYS:

- *LCHF diet causes weight loss and production of ketones which can treat pulmonary arterial hypertension (PAH).*
- *The anti-inflammatory effects of LCHF diet counteracts the inflammatory basis of PAH.*

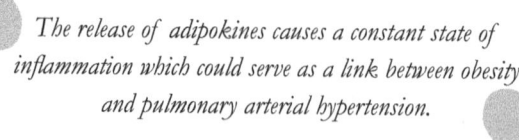

The release of adipokines causes a constant state of inflammation which could serve as a link between obesity and pulmonary arterial hypertension.

CHAPTER SIXTEEN

TREATMENT OF DIABETIC NEUROPATHY WITH LCHF DIET

CASE STUDY 7

The patient is a 48-year-old female, had DMT2 with severe diabetic neuropathy mainly peripheral, diagnosed clinically and by nerve stimulation.

Medications: Mixtard Insulin 26/16IU, and Pregabalin.

The patient was managed on a LCHF diet for 10 days and discharged on metformin.

The outpatient follow-up clinic showed a decreased HbA1c to 5.8 and mild Peripheral Neuropathy.

Discussion:
Peripheral neuropathy (PN) is nerve damage in a diabetic due to high blood sugar levels. Neuropathy can be peripheral; in feet, legs and hands or autonomic affecting organ functions e.g. digestive (gastropathy), urinary, temperature regulation, sexual function or cause postural hypotension. PN is an early complication of diabetes due to many years of hyperglycemia in DMT1 whereas in DMT2 it may be apparent after a few years of poor glycemic control or even at diagnosis.

A LCHF diet can potentially limit or reverse the progression of diabetic neuropathy. The diet helps to reduce blood sugar levels and the risk of neuropathy if good HbA1c can be achieved for many years; it also helps to reverse the symptoms of neuropathy although it has not been shown to reduce neuropathic pain.

Ketogenic diets and pain: A review article: Susan A Masino et al Trinity College (80). Ketogenic diet well established for anticonvulsant therapy is postulated to underlie pain and inflammation. A review of the clinical and basic

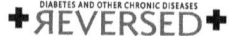

research of ketogenic diet (KD) on thermal and neuropathic pain and inflammation showed that KD can reduce inflammation and thus may be helpful in inflammation-associated pain. KD does not significantly affect neuropathic pain but reduces thermal pain.

Foot Care Education and tight stable glycemic control can lead to avoidance of foot ulcerations and amputations.

KEY TAKEAWAYS:
- *The LCHF diet leads to achieving good HbA1c and thus reduces the risk and prevents peripheral neuropathy*
- *There are many anecdotal reports of LCHF reversing or reducing focal, peripheral and autonomic neuropathy*

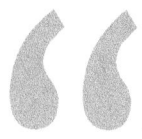

Foot Care Education and tight stable glycemic control can lead to avoidance of foot ulcerations and amputations.

Chapter Seventeen

TREATMENT OF CHRONIC PAIN SYNDROME e.g. SEVERE RHEUMATOID ARTHRITIS

This was a 62-year-old male, who was diagnosed with Severe Rheumatoid Arthritis (patient uses a wheelchair), Hypertension, and DMT2.

He was on Metformin and Glibenclamide, Non-steroidal anti-inflammatory agents (NSAIDs) and Losartan and amlodipine.

The patient was treated on a LCHF diet as an inpatient for 10 days and was discharged on metformin.

The Outpatient Clinic follow-up: anti-hypertensive medications were discontinued after 4 months.

After 6 months NSAIDs were withdrawn and the patient was on metformin only. This patient walks to the market and looks after his cattle.

Discussion:
Nine out of the 55 diabetic patients in our observational study had arthritis. The etiology of chronic pain syndrome (CPS) is very wide. It includes Rheumatoid Arthritis, Spinal Spondylosis, and Fibromyalgia. Rheumatoid arthritis and other Auto-Immune diseases can be additional comorbidity to diabetes. CPS can be due to general body inflammation **(80)**.

Inflammation: Peter Brunker: Professor Sports Medicine: **(81)** Outlines Inflammation (acute v/s chronic); what is a chronic disease? Role of Inflammation in chronic disease, can we measure inflammation, the role of diet in mediating inflammation.

Chronic inflammation is a common feature of most chronic diseases e.g. DMT2, Atherosclerosis, fibromyalgia, and chronic fatigue, Irritable Bowel Syndrome

(IBS), cancer, cardiovascular disease, autoimmune diseases, neurodegenerative diseases, mental illness e.g. depression, anxiety, etc.

63% of all deaths are due to non-communicable diseases and inflammation is a common factor in all these diseases. Markers of inflammation are non-specific and influenced by many factors but commonly used ones are hs-CRP and IL-6. Causes of inflammation include poor diet (sugar, processed foods, and vegetable oils), visceral obesity, lack of exercise, poor sleep, stress, alcohol, smoking, and lack of sun exposure.

Diet and relation to inflammation:

a) Carbohydrate and sugar: sweetened beverages, sweets, white bread intake is related to a rise in CRP and hs-CRP. Diet low in sugar and starch but high in fruit and vegetables leads to lower CRP and hs-CRP. There is no significant difference in hs-CRP between fructose and glucose. Persistent hyperglycemia due to carbohydrate intake increases inflammatory markers CRP etc. and reducing carbohydrates leads to a reduction in pro-inflammatory cytokines, chemokines, and adhesion molecules. High GI/GL foods increase chronic inflammatory markers. High fiber, whole grain is associated with reduced inflammation. Major flavonoids lower inflammation. Fruit polyphenols e.g. wine, berries, grapes, olive oil reduce inflammation.

b) It is not conclusive whether Saturated fats are inflammatory but polyunsaturated fats are inflammatory, omega 6 oils are inflammatory, omega 3 oils are anti-inflammatory; dairy is anti-inflammatory in patients with metabolic diseases and pro-inflammatory in subjects allergic to bovine milk.

c) Coffee, Black and green tea has no evidence of anti-inflammatory response found in cocoa (unsweetened).

d) Effects of diets on hs-CRP, Mediterranean, Tibetan, and DASH diets lead to significant CRP reduction, LCHF diets lead to a marked reduction in CRP. *Beta*-hydroxybutyrate (ketones) has an anti-inflammatory effect.

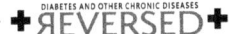

Vegan, vegetarian diets improve inflammation, especially after two years. Visceral inflammation occurs as a result of obesity.

Arthritis and weight loss: A case Study DR Doron Sher (Orthopedic Surgeon (82) discusses the case of a young overweight patient who needed surgery; had severe knee pain, treated with painkillers, physiotherapy, knee brace, and cortisone injections. Total Knee Replacement in obese patients takes longer, has more chance of DVT, a higher chance of infection and low satisfaction score, poor range of motion, more UTI, 5 times more chance of complications and device failure within 5 years. This is worse in diabetic patients whose obesity was due to Insulin Resistance. Blood tests show high HbA1c, CRP, ALT, TG, LDL, cholesterol, Creatinine, and low HDL. Mechanical stress contributes a lot to the development of osteoarthritis and obesity makes these stresses worse.

The metabolic causes of osteoarthritis are:
a) Low-grade inflammation; high CRP
b) Leptin
c) Omega 6 fatty acids
d) Matrix metalloproteinase (MMPS)
e) Hypertension
f) Diabetes
g) High abdominal circumference

The introduction of a LCHF diet led to diabetes remission, discontinuation of glycemic and blood pressure medications, weight loss, decrease in abdominal fat, LFTs and CRP. A 10% reduction in weight loss led to a 50% decrease in knee pain.

Low carb high-fat diet's fat loss helps to:
a) Reduce blood glucose level (less glycation improves tissue mechanics)
b) Reduce Omega 6's which reduce inflammation
c) Reduce MMPs which leads to 10% weight loss and 50% pain reduction and deferring or cancelation of the surgery
d) Reduce Inflammation; reduced medication use, improved exercise capacity, improved recovery
e) Improve mechanical loading.

*Investigating inflammation: DR Siobhan Huggins (83)*had signs of persistent inflammation, obesity, depression, acne, eczema, joint, and back pain before changing to a LCHF diet, and all these disappeared completely. Inflammation is associated with Auto-immune disorders e.g. Diabetes, Atherosclerosis, Alzheimer's disease, and Psoriasis. Acute inflammation has its purpose, to defend, repair and maintain tissues.

The functions of markers of acute inflammation are: Change in HDL function, high LDL particles, high VLDL/Triglycerides, higher lipoprotein (a), Insulin Resistance/hyperinsulinemia and high CRP.

Most of these are reflected in diabetes i.e. Low HDL, high triglycerides, high LDL-p, high CRP, Insulin Resistance/hyperinsulinemia, hyperglycemia and also in factors that increase CVD e.g. Diabetes, high CRP, high triglycerides, high blood pressure, low HDL, high lipoproteins, Insulin Resistance/hyperinsulinemia and high LDL-p. Therefore there is an overlap between acute and chronic inflammation. Chronic non-communicable diseases have acute inflammation all of the time, therefore remove the etiology causing the acute inflammation.

The ketogenic diet is anti-inflammatory that is why it is effective in the treatment of diabetes, autoimmune disorders, etc. Ketone bodies *Beta*-hydroxybutyrate (BHB) are directly anti-inflammatory.

*Can LCHF and ketogenic diets improve chronic pain? DR Evelyne Bourdua-Roy and DR Hala Lahlou: (84) Fam*ily *Physicians* share their clinical experience with LCHF ketogenic diet patients who had chronic pain associated with diabetes, and obesity, etc. which resolved with remission of these disorders.

Clinical chronic pain cases: Ankylosing spondylitis, back and knee pain due to osteoarthritis, fibromyalgia and irritable bowel syndrome, diabetes (with neuropathy and bilateral carpal tunnel syndrome, high CRP, depression); all lost some weight and their chronic pain improved.

Chronic pain definition, prevalence of associated comorbidities (e.g. obesity), impacts, treatment options, possible mechanisms through which ketogenic diets improve pain, (Mechanical-weight loss, the anti-inflammatory effect of ketone

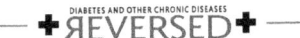
bodies, mitochondrial function and improved micronutrients): There are potential reasons for inflammation on Standard American Diet (SAD).

LCHF keto diets reduce Advanced Glycation End-products (AGES) leading to reduced inflammation and pain improvement.

Inflammation in the gut causes Crohn's disease, in the brain, Alzheimer's disease and in the nerves, increased Nociception and allodynia. Omega 6:3 ratio determines inflammation and LCHF ketogenic diets have a positive effect on inflammation since there is a reduction of omega 6 (vegetable oils) and increased intake of omega 3 rich foods.

Postprandial sugar spikes lead to CRP spikes and high GI and GL foods increase CRP.

Positive effects e.g. reduced pain is noted even in the absence of ketones in LCHF but being in ketosis results in better pain relief. Ketones improve pain signaling by anti-inflammatory effects, anticonvulsant effect, improved mitochondrial function and biogenesis, and adenosine signaling. The ketones through various pathways affect chronic pain threshold.

Micronutrients and pain:
   a) Vitamin D supplementation (50-70 U/kg/day) improves chronic pain especially in overweight (obesity) which is associated with vitamin D deficiency.
   b) Magnesium supplements 300-400 mg/day
   c) Other supplements that can ease chronic pain: omega 3, riboflavin, COQ10, cur cumin, glucosamine sulfate, probiotics, vitamin B1, B2, folate, calcium, amino acids, Zinc and Carnitine.

LCHF and ketogenic diets improve mood, attention and concentration, cognition and energy, leading to more motivation, less despair and hopelessness and decreased pain perception.

Obesity is associated with arthritis. Weight loss due to the LCHF diet leads to clinical improvement of arthritis and better inflammatory markers e.g. C-reactive protein (CRP).

Rheumatoid Arthritis (RA) can be treated with Dietary Intervention. LCHF diet helps in RA because it is anti-inflammatory, therefore it reduces symptoms and pain; causes relief from numbness, depression and weight loss in obesity associated with RA

Managing Rheumatoid Arthritis with Dietary interventions: Shweta Khanna et al (85)this article summarizes and discusses various diets that help in reducing levels of inflammatory cytokines in Rheumatoid arthritis (RA) that may play an effective role in the management of RA. An ideal meal can include raw or moderately cooked vegetables (lots of green vegetables and legumes) with the addition of spices like turmeric and ginger, seasoned fruits and probiotic yogurt.

Summary:
LCHF diet improves chronic pain by:
- Mechanical advantages e.g. weight loss
- Anti-inflammatory pathways LCHF diets decrease extrinsic and intrinsic Advanced Glycation End-products (AGES) which down-regulates inflammation and improves pain.
- Effect of ketone bodies: ketone bodies e.g. *beta*-hydroxybutyratedecrease inflammation.
- Effect of mitochondrial function: abnormal mitochondria in chronic pain are repaired leading to adenosine signaling.
- Improved micronutrient status, deficiency of vitamin D and Magnesium which lead to increased pain are improved by a LCHF diet.

KEY TAKEAWAYS:
- *The LCHF diet is anti-inflammatory and is useful in treatment of chronic pain syndromes and autoimmune diseases*
- *The LCHF diet causes weight loss, clinical pain improvement and better inflammatory markers e.g. CRP.*

CHAPTER EIGHTEEN

TREATMENT OF PROSTATE CANCER WITH LCHF DIET

CASE STUDY 9

The patient was a 77-year-old male confirmed to have prostate cancer after prostatectomy in 2012. He was on follow up with medications: Stilbestrol and bicalutamide (Casodex).

Orchidectomy was done in 2018.

In July 2019, he presented with nocturia, urine incontinence, abdominal pain, and gross hematuria. PSA was high. Pelvic X-Ray and pelvic ultrasound were done: nothing significant.

Diagnosis: Recurrent Prostate Cancer

Treatment: LCHF diet for 10 days as an inpatient
By the time the patient was discharged, he had no hematuria and urine incontinence had reduced.

Discussion:
The role of diet in the development and treatment of cancer requires larger trials but there is emerging evidence on the effectiveness of diet in the management of cancer. DMT2 patients have a high chance of developing cancer and exogenous insulin increases the growth of cancer. Insulin is a growth factor for Prostate cancer.

A LCHF diet causes a decrease in serum Insulin and Insulin-like Growth Factor 1 (IGF-1) and obesity leading to a decrease in cancer progression. LCHF diets target the Warburg effect in which cancer cells predominantly utilize glycolysis (burns glucose) instead of oxidative phosphorylation to produce ATP for energy. Thus, the rationale of the LCHF diet in cancer therapy is to reduce circulating levels of glucose and induce Nutritional Ketosis such that cancer cells are starved

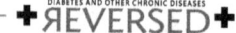
of energy while normal cells adapt their metabolism to use ketones (i.e. acetone, aceto-acetone, and *beta*-hydroxybutyrate) and survive.

Although larger trials are needed, data from case reports and trials suggest that LCHF diets are safe and tolerable for patients with cancer and may slow down prostate cancer growth.

Low carbohydrate diets and prostate cancer: How Low is Low Enough? Elizabeth M Masko et al (86)Prostate cancer is a common cancer worldwide. This study on mice fed on a No Carbohydrate Ketogenic Diet (NCKD) showed an increase in urinary ketones, decrease in the signaling of Insulin-like Growth Factor 1 (IGF-1) axis; a pathway known for progression of Prostate cancer but also well-known to be highly controlled through dietary intake leading to slowed tumor growth. To implement a no carbohydrate diet is difficult but patients can maintain in the long term a low carbohydrate diet e.g. Atkins since there is no difference between low carbohydrate and no carbohydrate diets in terms of prostate cancer growth and progression.

Examination of gene expression pattern in mitochondria and mutations in ketolytic and glycolytic enzymes may prove useful in selecting potentially responsive patients.

Ketogenic diets and Cancer: Emerging Evidence Jocelyn Tan-Shalaby (87)Gives mechanism of action of ketogenic diets and case reports. Recent study findings suggest KD is safe and tolerable for patients with cancer and combining Standard Chemotherapy and Radiotherapy may improve tumor response. Most Prostate cancers are not glycolytic but most recurrent cancers are glycolytic.

Is there a Role of a Low Carbohydrate Ketogenic Diet in the Management of Cancer? John C Mavropoulos et al (88) Low Carbohydrate Ketogenic Diet (LCKD) reduces serum Insulin levels. Insulin appears to play a role in Prostate cancer biology; reduced serum Insulin levels may be of clinical significance. Lower serum Insulin levels lower serum Insulin-like growth factor 1 (IGF-1) whose signaling pathway leads to a step in Prostate carcinogenesis. IGF-1 has been positively associated with Prostate cancer.

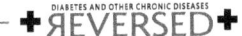
Tumor Metabolism and the Ketogenic Diets DR Andrienne Scheck (89)
Experimental protocol in rats shows that there is increased brain tumor survival of the ones on a ketogenic diet. Tumor radiated animals on ketogenic diets do better.

Pluripotent effects of Ketogenic Therapy:
- It reduces tumor growth
- It enhances Radiation and some Chemotherapies
- It reduces peritumoral oedema, inflammation, angiogenesis, hypoxia
- Expression of transcriptional activators
- Increases antitumor immune response.

Ketones recapitulate these effects in vitro in the absence of reduced glucose, *beta*-hydroxybutyrate (BHB) sensitizes cells to radiation by epigenetic alterations that affect gene expression; histone acetylation, non-coding RNAs, and alteration in DNA methylation. BHB radiosensitizes glioma stem cells. *Every hallmark of cancer is affected by the Ketogenic diet.*

Dietary Recommendations for Cancer/Warburg Metabolism: Clinical applications DR Colin Champ (90) Warburg Metabolism: DR Warburg 70 years ago found out that cancer cells rely on sugar through many metabolic pathways. Some cancer cells do not take glucose on the PET scan.

Blood glucose during treatment with KD: Glucose can be lowered with KD bringing better prognosis in Glioblastoma Multiforme (GBM). Patients with high fasting insulin have poorer prognosis e.g. Breast cancer, in such a case you can lower insulin through a ketogenic diet.

Dietary carbohydrate and IGF-1: High carbohydrate intake increases IGF-1; this puts patients at a higher risk of recurrence of breast cancer. In 1913 studies showed that more carbohydrate raises tumor growth in rats.

Meta-analyses of KD on cancer: Animal models show KD is preventative as well as treatment of cancer by itself or in combination with Chemotherapy and or Radiotherapy by lowering glucose level. Excess adipose tissue makes radiation less effective.

Insulin, glucose, and adipose tissue play an important role in tumor treatment and all these are positively affected by the LCHF ketogenic diet; e.g. weight gain, Metabolic Syndrome and Breast cancer recurrence relationship.

Cancer: Metabolic Disease with Metabolic Solutions: DR Thomas N Seyfield PhD (91) Incidence and deaths due to cancer are increasing. Current dogma is that cancer is a genetic disease; cancer cells carry the oncogenic and tumor suppressor mutation, and then define cancer as a genetic disease. Is there evidence that challenges the somatic mutation theory of cancer? Yes. Nuclear transplantation findings are incomparable with the somatic mutation theory of cancer.

Warburg Theory of Cancer (1956):
- Cancer arises from damage to cellular respiration.
- Energy through fermentation gradually decompensates for insufficient respiration.
- Cancer cells continue to ferment lactate in the presence of oxygen (Warburg effect).
- Enhanced fermentation is the signature metabolic malady of all cancer cells.

Therefore, cancer is a mitochondrial metabolic disease and calorie restriction (CR) is the metabolic cancer intervention since it:
a) Involves a total dietary intervention
b) Differs from starvation
c) Maintains mineral and nutrients
d) Enhances mitochondrial biogenesis and oxPhos
e) CR in mice mimics water only therapeutic fasting in humans.

Biomarkers of calorie restriction are:
- Reduce blood glucose.
- Elevate blood ketone levels.

Antitumor effects of calorie restriction are:
- Anti-angiogenic
- Anti-inflammatory
- Pro-apoptotic

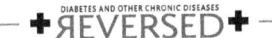
With the ketogenic diet, the same advantages of calorie restriction can be achieved. Composition of the Standard Diet (SD) and the Ketogenic diet

COMPONENT	STANDARD DIETS	KETOGENIC DIET
Carbohydrates	62	3
Fat	6	72
Proteins	27	15
Energy (Kcals/GM)	4.4	7.2
F/(P+C)	0.07	4

The ketogenic diet reduces blood glucose, elevates blood ketones and can provide long term management in inoperable brain tumors, Glioblastoma Multiforme (GBM) or recurrence.

The press pulse paradigm: A novel therapeutic strategy for the metabolic management of cancer involves Cyclic Energy Stress Targets mutated Tumor cells:

    a)   Calorie restricted Ketogenic diets } Press
    b)   Calorie restricted raw vegan diet } Press
    c)   Hyperbaric Oxygen Therapy } Pulse
    d)   Non-toxic drugs } Pulse

The glucose/ketone Index calculator is a simple tool to help manage cancer: *Glucose (Mmols/Ketone (Mmols) = Glucose Ketone Index (GKI).* Therapeutic efficacy is considered best with Index values approaching 1.0 or below.

Conclusion

    1. Preclinical and case report studies indicate that *the restricted metabolic Ketogenic diet (R-KD) can be an effective non-toxic "Metabolic Therapy" for managing malignant cancers in children and adults.*

    2. The therapeutic effects of the R-KD against cancer can be enhanced when combined with drugs or hyperbaric oxygen that also target energy metabolism; *'Press, Pulse' Paradigm.*

Ketogenic diet, Cancer metabolism, and the Warburg Effect: Prof Angela Poff (92) Though cancer can be due to genetic mutations, some cancers are due to derailed metabolic pathways that regulate energy; Warburg effect leading to a lot of glucose intake but lack of energy production. Cancer cells undergo fermentation process even in the presence of oxygen due to chromosomal dysfunction/abnormality in cancer cells leading to genetic mutations.

Hyperbaric oxygen improves oxygen supply to the tumor removing the signaling pathways created by tumor hypoxia. Hyperbaric oxygen is combined with the ketogenic diet. It also makes the tumor more susceptible to radiotherapy. Healthy mitochondria suppress cancer growth. This can be achieved by a well-formulated ketogenic diet.

Hyperglycemia and hyperinsulinemia are strong promoters of cancer growth. These are decreased by a ketogenic diet. Cancer thrives well in more oxidative stress; taking some antioxidants during chemotherapy or radiotherapy may reduce their effectiveness.

Ketones lower glucose and insulin but they also have separate gene signaling effects; they lower inflammation, reduce oxidative stress, inhibit glycolysis and reduce cancer cachexia. Ketogenic diet restores antitumor immunity.

LCHF (ketogenic) diet can be used as the:
a) Sole treatment with good results in some cancers e.g. Glioblastoma
b) Concurrently during Radiation and to enhance Chemotherapy
c) In advanced PET-positive tumors
d) In Cancer Cachexia with or without Sarcopenic Obesity.

Energy supply to a cancer can be reduced by moderate carbohydrate restriction, calorie reduction and intermittent fasting (IF).

Exploiting Cancer Metabolism with Ketosis and hyperbaric oxygen: Prof Angela Poff (93). Tumor cells rely on glucose, ketone bodies may have an anti-cancer effect in some tumors. They stimulate oxidative metabolism, inhibit inflammation, Histone Deacetylase Inhibitors (HDAC) inhibition, alter glycolysis, and reduce glucose. Ketones inhibit tumor growth and metastatic spread.

Combining metabolic therapies: hyperbaric oxygen

a) Hypoxia leads to tumor growth, aggressiveness, and metastasis and chemo radiation resistance.

b) Restoring oxygen may increase the sensitization of oxidative stress-mediated therapy e.g. Radiotherapy.

100% oxygen at elevated barometric pressure leads to elevated tissue partial pressure (Po2) leading to re-oxygenating hypoxic tumor cells. Combining KD and hyperbaric oxygen leads to the slowing of tumor growth.

Other cancer therapies:

- Modulating metabolism with glycemic agents
- Pharmacological Ascorbic acid
- Press Pulse Metabolic Therapy

The problem of cancer cachexia is highlighted.

Carbohydrate Restriction to Enhance Cancer Therapy: DR Dawn Lemmane (Integrative Medical Oncologist (94) "Healthy food for cancer patient according to American Cancer Society "snack often list." mTor plays a big role in cancer signaling growth. This signaling is related to Insulin and Insulin-like growth factor (IGF-1) and glucose/carbohydrate restriction.

Warburg effect: In a normal cell 1gram glucose molecule nets 38 ATP. In cancer with Warburg effect, 1 glucose molecule nets 2 ATP; therefore there are massive amounts of glucose needed to keep up with the energy demands. Cancer cells need 25 more glucose than normal cells.

Many cancers are etiologically unrelated to diet e.g.

- Pediatric cancers; most of these cancers can be cured with chemotherapy and diet is not the first choice of treatment
- Single chromosomal alteration e.g. Chronic Myeloid Leukemia (CML)
- Sarcoma
- HPV related cancers e.g. cervical, anal, vulvar, penile, throat, tongue
- EPV related cancers: Hodgkin's and non-Hodgkin's lymphoma
- Acute leukemia

Some cancers are seen in Diabetes e.g. Breast, pancreas, kidney, lung, stomach, prostate, uterus.

In DMT2 cancer risk is higher, cancer survival is lower and the data is consistent. Exogenous insulin is associated with increased cancer risk and decreased survival after diagnosis. Insulin increases the risk of cancer. Higher total and LDL cholesterol is associated with less incidence of certain cancers and better response to Chemotherapy and cancer-specific survival after diagnosis.

Triglyceride: HDL ratio (which is related to carbohydrate intake) predicts outcome in triple-negative breast cancer. The higher saturated fat intake, the better the prognosis. Higher cholesterol level is associated with decreased breast cancer incidence.

1. **Moderate carbohydrate restriction**: In Breast and colon cancer; in low carbohydrate (100gm per day) intake there is a better prognosis (mortality and recurrence). There is no connection between high-fiber, vegetables, low-fat, and breast cancer survival. In IGF-1 receptor-expressing breast cancers, decreasing carbohydrate was associated with better survival. Therefore moderate carbohydrate restriction is advised in Estrogen Responsive (ER) and postmenopausal breast cancer, and Stage III colon cancer if the patient is overweight. Start by restricting carbohydrates to 100gm per day, intermittent fasting (IF)/Caloric deficit is likely helpful.

2. **Ketogenic diet (KD):** Ketone bodies are *beta*-hydroxybutyrate, acetoacetate and acetone from fatty acids during fasting, prolonged exercise, and very low carbohydrate intake.

In ketogenic diet e.g. 85% fat, protein 10%, and carbohydrate 5%, measure ketosis by measuring blood ketones. KD has been used in refractory pediatric epilepsy.

Ketoacidosis is produced by an abnormal increase in blood ketones and uncontrolled DMT1, alcoholism, aspirin overdose and hyperemesis gravidarum. In ketoacidosis ketones are 15-25mmols/liter while in

Nutritional Ketosis levels are 0.5-5mmols/litre during ketogenic diets. A very low carbohydrate (ketogenic) diet does not cause ketoacidosis.

Glioblastoma multiforme (GBM) 5-year survival is zero but KD has promising results. Animal models show increased survival. Additional radiation increased survival. In radiation therapy, additional ketosis helps by lowering glucose levels which suppress angiogenesis. Low glucose decreases Insulin and IGF-1 signaling, decreases repair of radiation-induced DNA damage and decreases tumor regrowth, and therefore more radiation can be given without normal cell damage.

In cancer, cachexia is caused by inflammation and generalized inflammatory syndrome: Cytokines. Cancer cachexia is absent in early cancers (adjuvant setting), 2/3 of end-stage patients with solid tumors, weight loss more than 5%, BMI less than 20, and muscle wasting. One can be overweight or obese but have cancer cachexia e.g. Sarcopenic Obesity.

In certain tumors that have a mutation (BRAF VLODE) fat fuels tumor growth e.g. Some Melanomas, Leukemia, Colorectal cancer, Prostate cancer, and multiple myelomas. *Therefore test for it! These tumors may respond to statins.*

Summary:
Consider ketogenic diet during radiation, GMB, advanced PET-positive cancers, cancer cachexia, to enhance chemotherapy. Caution in BRAF VLODE.

Dietary suspects in cancer are fat, saturated fat, meat, dairy, carbohydrates, protein, specific amino acids, and cancer like food.

Some tumors use glucose and other energy sources e.g. fructose, lipids, choline, protein/amino acids (Glutamine, cysteine), acetate, and lactate. Therefore glutamine supplements may increase some tumor growth. Energy to tumors can be limited by calorie restriction, intermittent fasting, and longer fasts.

Chronic calorie restriction:
a) Cut daily calorie intake by 25-40%.
b) Delays degenerative diseases of aging (neurological, rheumatologic, malignant)

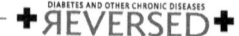

c) Extends life span in yeast, drosophila, vertebrates, and mammals
d) Underweight is a problem.

Intermittent fasting of 13-24 hours without calorie restriction lengthens lifespan even more than chronic restriction and maintains a normal weight. Intermittent fasting in consistent animal studies shows that it slows tumor growth (even without chemotherapy), potentiates chemotherapy and protects animal cells from treatment side effects. A 13-hour fasting 8 pm to 7 am is advised. Occasional 24-72 hour fasts may decrease cancer risk.

KEY TAKEAWAYS:

- *Some cancers are not diet related and respond well to chemotherapy and radiotherapy*
- *Some cancers respond better to LCHF diet than to chemotherapy and radiotherapy*
- *LCHF diet can be used as the sole treatment or concurrently with radiotherapy and chemotherapy in cancer treatment.*
- *Cancer cachexia is not a contraindication to LCHF diet*
- *Glucose Ketone Index (GKI) is a simple tool to help manage cancer*

> *The higher saturated fat intake, the better the prognosis. Higher cholesterol level is associated with decreased breast cancer incidence.*

CHAPTER NINETEEN

TREATMENT OF PSYCHIATRIC DISORDERS WITH LCHF KETOGENIC DIET

CASE STUDY 10

The patient was a 71-year-old Male with prediabetes, hypertension and panic disorder confirmed by a psychiatrist.

He had been on Irovel, Natrixam (indapamide), Arcalion (sulbutiamine), Biperiden HCL, Duloxetine, Loxiam MR, Etirocoxib, Haloperidol, Olanzapine and Risperidone.

The patient was admitted several times with temporary improvements, before the LCHF diet was started. Medications including antihypertensive agents were gradually withdrawn in 6 months. By the sixth month, the patient had lost 3kg and was in stable condition with LCHF and occasional carbohydrate recycling.

Discussion:

The role of Nutrition and or ketogenic diet in Psychiatry has not been widely studied. Studies done show that there is a relationship between diet and development and or treatment of Psychiatric disorders

Current Status of the Ketogenic diet (KD) in Psychiatry: Bostock E. C. et al (95) this review aimed to clarify the potential role of KD in psychiatry. The search yielded 15 studies related to the use of ketogenic diet in mental disorders including Anxiety, Depression, Bipolar disorder, and Schizophrenia, Autism Spectrum Disorder (ASD) and Attention Deficit Hyperactivity Disorder (ADHD). Nine were animal 4 case studies and 2 open-label studies in humans.

Results: reduced Depression-like behavior in rats, in bipolar; a reduction or no reduction in symptoms, Schizophrenia; reduced symptoms in two weeks of KD and ASD improvement.

Conclusion: The role of KD in mental disorders is unclear. There is insufficient evidence in humans. More studies are needed.

*Ketogenic Diets for Psychiatric Disorders: DR Georgia Ede: Psychiatrist (96)*Ketogenic diets have been used for many neurological disorders including epilepsy, metabolic disorders (obesity, etc.), cancer, DMT2, etc.

1. Ketogenic diets and bipolar II Disorder: KD was superior to lamotrigine in the management of symptoms.
2. KD and schizophrenia: positive outcomes
3. Ketogenic diets and anxiety: Reduced anxiety (animal studies).
4. Ketogenic diets and autism: Positive outcomes in animal models.
5. Ketogenic diets and ASD: Significant improvement in children.
6. KD and ADHD: Positive animal studies.

More human studies needed.

KD and Psychiatric Medications: DR Georgia Ede: Psychiatrist: (97) "Ketogenic diets cause profound shifts in brain and body chemistry rather quickly and the changes have a major impact on medication levels, dosages, and side effects and require close medical supervision, particularly in the first month or two while your metabolism adjusts to your new healthy way of eating.

Before you start a low carbohydrate/KD for mental health purposes:
a) Discuss the idea with the psychiatrist/psychiatric nurse who prescribes your medications first before making any changes to your diet.
b) Your prescribing clinician should be supportive and knowledgeable about ketogenic diets or be ready to cooperate with other health professionals who can guide them.
c) Do some blood tests
   I) Fasting Comprehensive Metabolic Panel (glucose, electrolytes, kidney function, liver function, and acid-base balance).
   II) Fasting Lipid Panel including HDL cholesterol and triglycerides.
   III) Fasting Total Insulin Level.
   IV) Any relevant medication levels e.g. Lithium and Depakote.

V) Any other tests recommended.

d) Blood pressure, heart rate, BMI, and waist circumference.

e) Follow up appointments; weekly, in the first 4-6 weeks.

Mental health patients with insulin resistance benefit more from KD.

After the first 6 weeks, the clinician should consider any medication reductions. Never stop any medications abruptly! Always the clinician should taper down very slowly and change only one medication at a time! Remember it can take up to 6 weeks for brain effects of most psychiatric effects to completely reverse them. Wait at least 6 weeks between each medication taper.

On starting KD diet side effects may be felt in the first few days e.g. irritability, mood swings, sleep changes and cravings.

1. **Antipsychotic medications and Ketogenic diets:** Antipsychotic medications e.g. Resperidal can increase insulin level and cause insulin resistance; make it difficult to achieve Nutritional Ketosis and have to be lowered or gradually stopped for full ketosis to be realized.

2. **Lithium and KD:** KD leads to diuresis, therefore, the concentration of lithium in the blood increases leading to increased side effects which may necessitate dosage downward adjustment. Replacing lost salts e.g. Magnesium and potassium is essential.

3. **Anticonvulsant mood stabilizers and KD**: These medications are prescribed for mood disorders e.g. Depakote (Valproate) which is a fatty acid burned by the body for fuel, therefore blood levels of Depakote may fall; this may require increasing the dose temporarily.

Zonisamide and Topiramate (anticonvulsants) cause metabolic acidosis and therefore increase the risk of kidney stones together with a KD.

4. **Blood pressure medications** may need to be adjusted e.g. clonidine, prazosin, propranolol also used in insomnia, anxiety, nightmares, and ADHD.

5. **Constipation and psychiatric medications**: KD and psychiatric medications can cause constipation.

6. **Other health conditions and non-psychiatric medications**: Check with your clinician.

NB. If you are taking psychiatric medications, educate yourself, plan; work closely with your mental health provider before embarking on a ketogenic diet.

Ketogenic Diet as a Metabolic Therapy for Mood Disorders: Evidence and Developments: Brutzke et al (98) despite significant advances in pharmacological and non-pharmacological treatments, mood disorders remain a significant source of treatment of mental capital loss with high rates of treatment resistance. KD is an effective anticonvulsant and has profound effects on multiple targets implicated in the pathophysiology of mood disorders including glutamate/GABA transmitters, monoamine levels, mitochondrial function and biogenesis, neurotrophism, oxidative stress, insulin dysfunction, and inflammation.

Preclinical studies, case reports, and case series have demonstrated antidepressant and mood-stabilizing effects of KD but to date, no clinical trials for depression or bipolar have been conducted. KD should be considered as a promising intervention in mood disorder therapeutics.

James R Phelps et al: The ketogenic diet for type-2 bipolar Disorder: (99). Successful mood-stabilizing treatments reduce intracellular Sodium in an activity-dependent manner. This can be achieved with acidification of the blood as it is the case with the ketogenic diet.

Two women with Type-2 Bipolar disorder were able to maintain ketosis for prolonged periods (2 and 3 years respectively). Both experienced mood stabilization that exceeded that achieved with medication; experienced a subjective improvement that was distinctively related to ketosis; and tolerated the diet well. There were no significant adverse effects in either case. These cases demonstrate that the ketogenic diet is a potentially sustainable option for mood stabilization in type-2 Bipolar illness. They also support the hypothesis that acidic plasma may stabilize mood, perhaps by reducing intracellular Sodium and Calcium.

Dr. Georgia Ede: *The brain needs meat: mental benefits of the carnivorous diet:* **(100)** it is remarkable that studies of truly indigenous populations are virtually unanimous in reporting a very low rate of schizophrenia". The dietary root causes of mental illness are related to deficiency, toxicity, and metabolic mayhem.

1. **Nutrient deficiency**: the brain contains fat, protein, cholesterol, micronutrients, glucose or ketones for energy. Common deficiencies of zinc, vitamin B6, iron, vitamin D, B12, Magnesium, Omega 3 fatty acids affect various brain functions.

Meat has very essential micronutrients while plants lack some essential micronutrients. Plants are low in Carnitine and Choline. Carnitine is essential for the balance of brain energy/tonicity while Choline is essential for cell integrity and acetylcholine synthesis.

Cholesterol cannot cross the blood-brain barrier; the brain makes its own. Animal proteins are more complete, offer most proteins per ounce, most digestible, bioavailable and have no anti-nutrients.

The brain is 60% fat, Omega 3(DHA) plays a unique and indispensable role in the neural signaling essential for higher intelligence, this is mainly got from animal and very hard to extract from plant foods.

Animal meat eaters have higher levels of Eicosapentaenoic acid (EPA) and DHA than vegetarians and vegans. Arachidonic acid (ARA), an omega 6 fatty acid is usedfor many body functions but is also involved in inflammation which is important in repair and healing.

ARA is mainly from animal foods; the brain needs meat, it does not have to be red meat, poultry or fish.

2. Toxicity in psychiatric diseases: Plant toxins affect the brain; glycoalkaloids, oxalates, lectins, gluten. People with schizophrenia,

bipolar disorder and autism spectrum disorders (ASD) are more likely to have antibodies to gluten (wheat) and casein derived peptides (milk). Up to 70% of ASD have markers of leaky gut.

Some patient's schizophrenia responds to a gluten-free diet. In leaky gut, toxins can affect the brain directly through the vagus nerve or indirectly through inflammatory messengers that cross into the brain.

In plant-based logic, there is demonization of nutrient e.g. heme iron causes iron overload and colon cancer, Carnitine causes heart disease via Trimethylamine N-Oxide(TMAO), arachidonic acid causes inflammation, cholesterol causes heart disease and glorification of (PI) antinutrients e.g. phytic acid (grains/beans/nuts/seeds), sulfoxone (garlic, onions, leeks), fiber (all plants), sulforaphane (crucifers).

3. Metabolic mayhem: involves inflammation and oxidation, neurotransmitter imbalances, and Insulin Resistance e.g. lowering Insulin level by LCHF and improving your Metabolic Health.

Depression and bipolar disorder are linked to inflammation. Depression, bipolar disorder, Schizophrenia, Developmental Coordination Disorder (DCD) is linked to oxidation.

Neurotransmitter imbalances can be linked to mental health e.g. serotonin (depression), dopamine/psychosis (ADHD), glutamate/GABA (overall activity level of the brain).

Processed and seed foods are a common cause of oxidation and inflammation stress leading to 100 times more glutamine leading to an imbalance of dopamine, GABA, and other transmitters and brain damage.

Glutamine decreases BDNF (neuroplasticity); how the brain recovers from stress, shrinks the hippocampus, injures proteins, lipids, DNA, mitochondria, and damages the blood-brain barrier.

Insulin resistance and Psychosis: people diagnosed with schizophrenia are more likely to have glucose regulation problems and insulin resistance even if they have never taken antipsychotic medications.

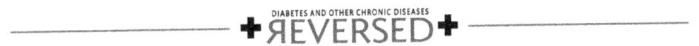
Insulin resistance and Bipolar: Patients with bipolar disorder type-1 and 2 and insulin resistance are more likely to be chronically symptomatic, rapid cycling and lithium refractory (BMI predictive).

Insulin resistance and depression: Treating the insulin resistance and some anti-inflammatory medications improves depression in 7 out of 8 studies.

Epilepsy is treatable with the ketogenic diet. Bipolar disorders and epilepsy are connected therefore seizure medications are used to treat bipolar disorder.

Ketogenic diet and mood stabilizer medications lower sodium inside brain cells. Therefore ketogenic diets and ketosis could be helping in glutamate dysregulation, mitochondrial dysfunction, oxidative stress, excess inflammation, serotonin deficit, and low BDNF. A ketogenic diet could help in Parkinson's disease, ALS, traumatic brain injury, multiple sclerosis, epilepsy, autism, and bipolar disorder, psychosis, and Alzheimer's disease.

A carnivore diet may be suitable for mental health because some people have lost the ability to manage plant toxins.

Carnivore and vegan are both extreme diets but vegan diets are bio-illogical.

In 2017 Bostock review clinical improvements were noted in some patients on LCHF diets with anxiety, depression, Bipolar disorder, and schizophrenia (**95**)

Other psychiatric patients whose condition improves LCHF diet Bulimia and Attention Deficit Hyperactivity Disorder (ADHD). Care should be taken since the LCHF diet is contraindicated in some eating disorders e.g. Anorexia Nervosa.

The initiation of a LCHF diet in a psychiatric patient protocol includes

    a)   Metabolic profile: urea and electrolytes (U/E), lipid profile, blood pressure (B/P), heart rate, weight, etc. insulin medications, blood medication levels e.g. lithium; LCHF diet can change blood levels of lithium.

    b)   Careful follow-up and gradual withdrawal of medications

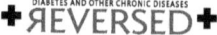

KEY TAKEAWAYS:

- *Diet has a role in the management of psychiatric illnesses.*
- *Psychiatric disorders are related to nutrients and brain neurotransmitters*
- *The LCHF diet can counteract some side effects of psychotropics e.g. Weight gain*

> *Animal proteins are more complete, offer most proteins per ounce, most digestible, bioavailable and have no anti-nutrients.*

CHAPTER TWENTY

TREATMENT OF OBESITY WITH LCHF DIET

CASE STUDY 11

The patient is a 61-year-old male; he was diagnosed with DMT2, hypertension, diabetic foot, severe Rheumatoid Arthritis, and Obesity.

This is the same patient in case study number 1. His DMT2, Hypertension, Severe Rheumatoid Arthritis, and obesity were controlled using the LCHF diet. Within 8 months, his weight decreased from 110Kg to 72 Kg and within one year on the LCHF diet, he was still maintaining a normal BMI.

Discussion:
Various studies have demonstrated the effectiveness of the LCHF diet in weight reduction in obese patients. The diet is safe and effective in the long term. It significantly reduces body weight and body mass index (BMI), decreases triglyceride, LDL Cholesterol, and blood glucose and increases HDL Cholesterol

Long Term Effects of a Ketogenic Diet in Obese Patients: Hussein M Dashti et al (101). Although various studies have examined the short term effects of a ketogenic diet in reducing weight in obese patients, its long-term effects on various physical and biochemical parameters are unknown. The objective of this study was to determine the effect of a 24-week ketogenic diet in obese patients. The study showed beneficial effects of a long term ketogenic diet; it significantly reduced the body weight and body mass of the patients, decreased blood glucose, triglycerides, and LDL cholesterol and increased HDL cholesterol. No significant side effects were noted and therefore the study confirms that it is safe to use the ketogenic diet for a longer period than previously demonstrated.

Optimal management of overweight and obese patients requires an emphasized combination of diet, exercise, and behavioral change.

DR Lucy Burns: The hormonal approach to obesity (102) Obesity is a global epidemic. The battle is the sheer number of people who are obese, to bring up the topic without offense, marketing giants who send mixed messages on the health of their products, the addictive nature of hyper-palatable foods and obesogenic environment, poor nutritional science, and low quality studies, and Medicare: current model rewards high through-put medicine.

Diet and exercise do not work. Obesity is hormonal, and not a calorie problem. Long term low calorie diet does not work. Major hormones involved in obesity are Insulin, Glucagon, Incretin, and Glucagon-like Peptide-1 /Gastric Inhibitory Polypeptide (GLP-1/GIP), Leptin, Ghrelin, Peptide YY and Adiponectin.

Side players: Cortisol, estrogen, progesterone, thyroid hormone, nutritional deficiencies, gut microbiome, and drugs (Insulin, prednisolone, antipsychotics). Insulin is the Master hormone. It maintains glucose between 4-5.5mmols/Litre, facilitates glucose uptake into muscle, liver and fat cells, inhibits glycolysis (the breakdown of glycogen), and inhibits lipolysis (stops fat breakdown) that makes patients who are on exogenous Insulin to gain weight.

Plan for Weight Loss: this includes 8 sessions 40minutes each individual/ group or online. Two sessions are on diet and pathology e.g. Insulin, 4 are on the psychological aspect of obesity, one on gut health and one on intermittent fasting.

A. Diagnose the problem: Insulin Resistance
1. Weigh the patient
2. Take waist circumference >88cm for women and >102cm for men
3. HbA1c (>5.5)
4. Homa IR
5. Glucose Tolerance Test (GTT) with corresponding Insulin levels and Kraft test; this is the definitive test of Insulin resistance. Kraft Test is a GTT with corresponding Insulin levels for earlier diagnosis of diabetes and enables us to diagnose diabetes much earlier than we do.

Diabetes is a vascular disease and abnormal Insulin levels damage the vascular system in every body organ.

High Insulin (hyperinsulinemia) is the causal mechanism behind most metabolic and chronic diseases today e.g. CVD, CVA, DMT2, NAFL, Osteoarthritis, hypertension, PCOS, Inflammation, and obesity.

NB. In Kraft curves, normal FBS, and HbA1c are normal after carbohydrate challenge but insulin remains high on GTT, therefore there is a feeling of hunger and another bout of eating.

Hyperinsulinemic patient has a lot of fat stores which he cannot access and therefore he gets hungry and has to eat more.

Carbohydrates stimulate more insulin production than proteins and fats, to reduce insulin reduce dietary carbs then the pancreas won't have to produce large amounts of Insulin. This is achieved by giving a LCHF diet as the first step; fish, eggs, etc. Whole foods. Carbs are addictive and patients don't leave them easily.

A. **Work on the psychological issues of the patient**

B. **Sleep:** Sleep increases Insulin Resistance. Short sleep duration is associated with reduced Leptin, elevated Ghrelin and increased Body Mass Index (BMI), weakens resolve, and increases emotional eating.

C. **Gut Health:** Remove any potential triggers of inflammation, remove any foods that may increase intestinal permeability, wheat, leptins, dairy A1 Protein, increase probiotics, recommend food/diet change.

D. **Intermittent fasting: IF** leads to reduced Insulin Resistance and increases autophagy.

E. **Have support groups** e.g. Facebook group, evening session, monthly session for those who have completed the program and long term behavioral changes.

KEY POINTS
1. A vast majority of people with obesity are Insulin resistant.
2. Diagnose and document the condition.

3. Obesity is a disease process that is both the result of and the cause of hormonal derangement.
4. Obesity is an inflammatory process.
5. It is treatable.
6. It requires dietary and lifestyle interventions and long-term behavioral changes.
7. Change is possible.

Adherence not diet type is more important in sustaining weight loss. Calories in, calories out (CICO) does not work. We have to understand the psychophysiological cycle of obesity and treat obesity as a substance (Carbohydrate) abuse and therefore use addiction principles to treat obesity.

Sugar Addiction: Is it real? Divicolantonio et al (103) in animal studies sugar has been found to produce more symptoms than it is required to be considered an addictive substance. In humans, there is substantial parallel and overlap between drugs of abuse and sugar.

Sugar addiction: The State of the Science: Westwater M. L. et al (104) as obesity rates continue to rise; the notion that overconsumption reflects underlying food addiction has become increasingly influential. An increasingly popular theory is that sugar acts as an addictive agent similar to drug addiction. This paper reviews the evidence in support of sugar addiction.

The suggested mechanism of weight reduction with LCHF diet can be due to reduction in appetite, reduction in lipogenesis, increased lipolysis and increased metabolic cost of gluconeogenesis and thermic effect of proteins, changes in hormones of ghrelin and leptin, which control appetite (78)

*Eric Westman, William Yancy et al: Use of a low carbohydrate Ketogenic diet to treat Obesity (105)*Points that obesity prevalence is reaching pandemic levels in the USA 40% and worldwide. Ketogenic diets have been under increased scientific scrutiny and acceptance since 1863. The low carb diets can be combined with intermittent fasting and advantages include reduction of hunger, improved serum triglyceride, and LDL which is associated with a reduction in cardiovascular risk and greater glycemic control.

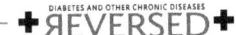
Side effects include mild fatigue, headache, diarrhea, constipation and muscle cramps. This article gives a detailed explanation of the use of the ketogenic diet for a successful and sustainable weight loss in the treatment of obesity. It covers instruction/monitoring of a KD, medical evaluation before the use of a KD, examples of foods allowed on the diet, follow-up and medical evaluation, deprescribing of medications, side effects, and their treatment.

Masood W et al: "In Ketogenic diet" (106) concludes that a very low carb high fat (VLCHF) ketogenic diet has proved to be very effective for rapid sustained weight loss.

"Dietary treatment for obesity by Peter M Clifton (107): Discusses carbohydrate-restricted diets and shows that carbohydrate-restricted weight-loss diets with a modest increase in protein intake can have beneficial effects on weight and lipids compared with high carb diets and this benefit can persist for as long as two years.

In a randomized trial of *a low carbohydrate diet v/s orlistat plus a low-fat diet for weight loss Yancy W S et al 2010 Arch. Intern. Med*, two groups of overweight patients with obesity-associated diabetes, high blood pressure, high cholesterol, and arthritis. The low carb group had the same weight loss (10%), 47% compared to 27%, blood pressure decreased or discontinued, more drop in systolic blood pressure, equal drop in cholesterol and glucose drop than the orlistat (a weight-loss drug) group.

Conclusion
For people with high blood pressure and a weight problem, a low carb diet might be a better option than a weight loss medication. Low carb diet gives the same weight loss with fewer costs and potentially lower side effects.

KEY TAKEAWAYS:
- *Obesity is a hormonal problem*
- *The LCHF diet causes sustained weight loss than low-calorie diets.*
- *Addiction principles should be applied in treatment of obesity*

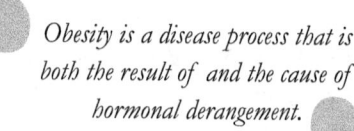

Obesity is a disease process that is both the result of and the cause of hormonal derangement.

CHAPTER TWENTY ONE

TREATMENT OF NEURODEGENERATIVE DISEASES: (ALZHEIMER'S/PARKINSON'S etc.) WITH LCHF DIET

CASE STUDY 12

The patient was an 86-year-male; he was diagnosed with DMT2, Alzheimer's disease, and hypertension.

He was on Losartan H, Mixtard insulin 35/15 IU. On admission, the patient was managed on soluble insulin (PRN), LCHF diet including MCT coconut oil.

After a 10-day admission, there was a great improvement in memory and was discharged on Metformin and Losartan H.

Discussion:
Alzheimer's disease (AD); the leading cause of Dementia among the aged is known to be associated with diabetes and is commonly known as Diabetes Type 3 (DMT3). The etiology includes insulin resistance, therefore the association between Alzheimer's disease AD and DMT2. The reversal of DMT2 leads to improvement and or slow progression of AD.

Can Ketone Bodies Slow down Alzheimer's disease? Stephen Cunnane (108)
Pioneers include Miia Kivipetto who demonstrated that 'prevention' works to slow down cognitive decline in older people. (The Finger Trial; Lancet 2015).

The brain runs on glucose and ketones (acetone, acetoacetate and betahydroxybutyrate) from dietary or stored fatty acids. If the brain glucose goes down, ketones enter the brain i.e. Brain Energy Metabolism depends on 2 distinctly different strategies for the 2 main fuels; glucose is pulled into the cell while ketones are pushed into the brain when they go up in the blood. The infant's brain is constantly using ketones mainly from the milk. Ketones are the brain's preferred fuel in healthy adults in short term Nutritional Ketosis.

In Alzheimer's disease, there is *glucose hypo hypometabolism* mainly in parietal lobes. Lowered brain energy precedes a cognitive decline in conditions associated with increased risk of Alzheimer's disease. This is called *Latent Pre-symptomatic Brain Glucose hypo Metabolism* in older people, in insulin resistance, family history of Alzheimer's, ApoE4 carrier, presonillin-1, and in regional deficit (8-10%) is lower than young healthy adults. This leads to neuropathology. The deterioration of synapses, brain structure, and function leads to cognitive decline and the vicious cycle of brain energy exhaustion and the progression of Alzheimer's disease. The brain cell is not dying because it has no glucose uptake but has low ketone uptake. The brain in Alzheimer's disease (AD) increases uptake of ketones when they are available depending on plasma levels.

Tests for cognitive impairment show improvement after 6 months on MCT oil in Mild Cognitive Impairment (MCI).

Other clinical studies on the ketogenic diet and MCT oil in patients with Alzheimer's showed the same results depending on the brain energy gap in MCI.

In diabetes type-2, Insulin resistance (IR) prevents ketones and glucose entry into the brain cell. This IR in young women with polycystic ovary syndrome (PCOS) causes mild defects in working memory although BMI is normal.

In a clinical *Trial by Miia Kivipelto*: Finish Neurologist KETO FINGER TRIAL which included:
1. Physical activity 3 times a week.
2. Cardiometabolic risk reduction (lower insulin levels).
3. Cognitive and social stimulation (Use of computers together).
4. Better Nutrition.
5. Added ketogenic supplements.

All the above resulted in an improvement in MCI.

Exogenous ketone salts and MCT oils supplements slowed Alzheimer's disease progression.

Metformin decreases insulin resistance and can help in Alzheimer's disease.

Unconventional but Effective Therapy for Alzheimer's disease: DR Mary Newport (109) explains her husband's cognitive decline due to Alzheimer's disease now known as Type 3 Diabetes due to Insulin resistance which makes the brain cells unable to use glucose.

Ketogenic diets produce ketones which offer an alternative brain fuel source. Medium-chain triglycerides (MCTs) are also used to produce ketones in the liver. MCT oil is extracted from coconut.

She started her husband on coconut oil; 7teaspoonfuls with breakfast. His Mini-Mental State Exam (MMSE) scale improved. MCT oil produces more ketones than coconut oil. She was mixing MCT and coconut oil and gradually decreased the dose. His MMSE scale kept on improving drastically. She started publicizing her husband's improvement of Alzheimer's on coconut/MCT oils, and subsequently wrote a book *"Alzheimer's: What if there was a 'cure'.* This has led to the development of exogenous ketone esters.

Alzheimer's disease: Type 3 Diabetes: Amy Berger (KETOCON 2018) (110) starts with Alzheimer's disease: (AD) statistics. AD is a metabolic Disease; the brain is an energy hog but in AD there is a reduction in glucose metabolism and mitochondrial dysfunction. The neurons have decreased glucose metabolism due to Insulin resistance and hyperinsulinemia. Therefore, it is referred to as diabetes type 3. AD is progressive even from an early age. The APOE4 gene is associated with AD but not the cause. Amyloid plaques accumulate because they are not being cleared and it's not the cause of AD. The drugs aimed at reducing the plaques do not positively affect disease progression. Amyloid may be protective of brain cells aiming to reduce oxidative stress. Under hyperinsulinemic conditions, Insulin competes with amyloids for Insulin Degrading Enzyme (IDE) leading to plaque formation.

Statins contribute to Dementia and Cognitive decline. High cholesterol is associated with better cognitive function in the elderly.

Ketones are used as preferred fuel by the brain instead of glucose. Ketone levels can be raised by a low carbohydrate/ketogenic diet, fasting, exercise, coconut oil and or MCT oil and exogenous ketones.

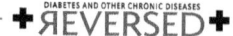
Alzheimer's disease can be prevented through nutrient-dense Low-carbohydrate low Insulin stimulating diets.

Ketogenic Diets and Alzheimer's disease: Klaus w Lange et al (111) Alzheimer's disease (AD) is a progressive neurodegenerative disease characterized by a decline in cognitive function and associated with amyloid plaques and neurofibrillary tangles.

There is progressive cerebral glucose hypo metabolism; ketones bodies produced during glucose deprivation can supplement the glucose.

This review provides a synopsis of clinical trials assessing the efficacy of ketogenic diets in the treatment of Alzheimer's disease. Both exogenous ketones and low carbohydrate high-fat diets are efficacious in clinical studies with AD patients.

The Role of Ketogenic diets in Neurodegenerative diseases (Alzheimer's disease/Parkinson's disease): Darusz Włodarek et al (112) the goal of this review was to assess the effectiveness of ketogenic diet (KD) on the therapy of neurodegenerative diseases. The KD is a Low carbohydrate High-Fat diet (LCHF) which results in Nutritional Ketosis. It has been used in resistant epilepsy for over 100 years but current studies indicate possible neuroprotective effects. Only a few studies have evaluated the role of KD in the prevention of Parkinson's and Alzheimer's diseases.

Some studies have demonstrated reduction of the disease symptoms but KD in the elderly may have special challenges e.g. reduced appetite may lead to Malnutrition and long-term effects of the KD in patients with these neurodegenerative diseases needs further research.

The underlying pathology of AD is not yet fully understood but it could be related to amyloid plaques which accumulate in the brains of patients with AD; impaired glucose metabolism and neural cell death. LCHF diet could alleviate the effects of impaired glucose metabolism by providing ketones as a supplementary source of energy to reduce the accumulation of amyloid plaques. The ketogenic diet is antioxidant and anti-inflammatory and can be a new perspective for Neuro-protection in AD.

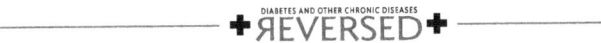
Ketogenic diet in Alzheimer's disease: Review: Marta Rusek et al (113) "The prevalence of Alzheimer's disease (AD) is increasing; the pathology could be deposition of amyloid plaques and impaired glucose metabolism. Dietary interventions could target these issues. Ketogenic diet through the production of ketone bodies can play a potential role in AD progression and its implementation can be a therapeutic strategy for Alzheimer's disease.

KEY TAKEAWAYS:

- *Alzheimer's disease is commonly known as Diabetes type-3 and is mainly due to insulin resistance*
- *The LCHF diet is an unconventional but effective therapy for Alzheimer's disease*
- *The ketones due to LCHF diet treat and prevent Alzheimer's and Parkinson's disease*
- *MCT oil and coconut oil augment the effects of LCHF diet in Alzheimer's disease.*

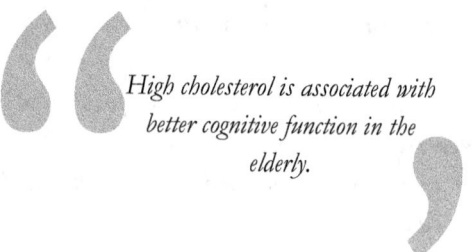

> *High cholesterol is associated with better cognitive function in the elderly.*

CHAPTER TWENTY TWO

TREATMENT OF CEREBROVASCULAR ACCIDENT (CVA) WITH LCHF DIET

CASE STUDY 13 A AND B

We had four (4) CVA patients in our observational study; one patient had Thrombotic CVA not associated with DMT2 or hypertension, two patients had CVA associated with DMT2 and Hypertension and one patient had Hypertensive CVA.

A. Hypertensive CVA case

This was a 45-year-old male; with severe Hypertensive stroke confirmed by Brain CT SCAN. He was managed on Enalapril, Losartan, hydralazine, and Atenolol.

Motor power improved from grade-1 to grade-4 in 9 days on a LCHF diet plus physiotherapy and antihypertensive medications.

The patient was discharged on Losartan.

B. Thrombotic CVA case not associated with DMT2 or hypertension

The patient was a 55-year-old male; had febrile illness; elevated White Blood Cells (WBCs) and was treated with antibiotics. Meningitis was ruled out.

The patient presented with sudden onset of thrombotic stroke which was confirmed by a Brain CT SCAN.

Management: LCHF diet, fluoxetine, clopidogrel.

He was discharged on low dose Aspirin and LCHF diet

After 3 months of follow-up there was no change in motor function from grade 1. Case A responded well to a LCHF diet, antihypertensive medications, and Physiotherapy.

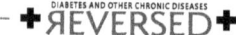
Case B: Thrombotic stroke did not have a remarkable improvement in motor function after three months of LCHF diet, anticoagulants and Physiotherapy.

Discussion:
Arterial occlusion disrupts glucose and oxygen supply in a clinical area of the Brain resulting in Ischemic Stroke characterized by excitotoxicity, oxidative stress, and apoptosis. A LCHF (ketogenic) diet results in increased ketone production. The ketones are used by the brain as an alternative energy source instead of glucose just like in neurodegenerative conditions e.g. Alzheimer's, Parkinson's disease, etc. The diet reduces excitotoxicity, oxidative stress, and apoptosis leading to healing of remaining neurons in the penumbra zone.

*Ketogenic Diet provides Neuroprotective Effects against Ischemic Stroke Neural Damages: Sheida Shaafi et al (114)*Ischemic stroke is a worldwide leading cause of death and disability. The ketogenic diet has been used successfully in epilepsy and other neurological disorders. It is postulated that a ketogenic diet through ketone bodies could provide benefit to the treatment of cerebral ischemic injuries through the following mechanisms:

a) Regulates excitotoxicity
b) Reduction of oxidative stress
c) Reduction of apoptosis.

The diet also reduces brain inflammation after traumatic brain injury since it is anti-inflammatory.

Inflammation after Stroke or Traumatic Brain injury: Jack Woodfield (115)
Ketogenic diet could reduce inflammation after a stroke or brain injury. Animal models show that a ketogenic diet suppresses the activity of inflammatory genes.

KEY TAKEAWAYS:
- *LCHF diet reduces brain inflammation after stroke or traumatic brain injury.*
- *The LCHF diet can be neuroprotective in ischaemic stroke.*

CHAPTER TWENTY THREE

TREATMENT OF DIABETIC NEPHROPATHY AND RETINOPATHY WITH LCHF DIET

CASE STUDY 14

The patient was an 80-year-old male, diagnosed with diabetes 20 years prior. He had very poor vision and used a walking stick, had leg edema, high B/P, swollen joints, abdominal discomfort, and vomiting.

Diagnosis: DMT2, hypertension, diabetic retinopathy and nephropathy, severe arthritis, diabetic Gastropathy, and Peripheral neuropathy

Medications:
He was on 15 different types of medications including Mixtard insulin 30/20 IU, metformin, furosemide 80mg BD, Methyldopa 500mg BD, Hydralazine 50mg TDS, Low dose Aspirin, Atorvastatin, etc. The patient was started on a LCHF diet, Mixtard insulin injection was stopped immediately and was put on Soluble Insulin PRN; other medications were withdrawn gradually.

The patient was discharged on Metformin, low doses of methyldopa, hydralazine, and furosemide.

Follow up: Vision had remarkably improved; no leg edema, maintaining normal B/P with methyldopa, hydralazine reduced doses; reduced joint pain and he could walk without support/aid.

HbA1c dropped from 10.3 to 6.5, Urea and electrolyte/creatinine (UECs) markedly improved. He lost 2Kg and felt mentally alert.

Discussion:
This case study shows the benefits of the LCHF diet for patients with DMT2 for a long duration with multiple diabetic complications. He managed to reduce weight, lower HbA1c, reverse nephropathy, retinopathy, gastropathy, hypertension and arthritis/gout. *This implies that it is never too late for a patient*

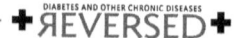
to benefit from a LCHF diet and for medications to be gradually reduced with an accompanying reduction in the severity of diabetic complications **(50).** The reversal of diabetic nephropathy has been well documented.

Reversal of Diabetic Nephropathy by a ketogenic diet: Poplawski et al (116)Diabetic nephropathy as indicated by albumin/creatinine ratios, as well as expression of stress-induced genes, was completely reversed by 2 months maintenance on a ketogenic diet. However, histological evidence of nephropathy was only partially reversed.

These studies demonstrate that diabetic nephropathy can be reversed by a relatively simple dietary intervention.

Diabetic retinopathy (DR) is a major micro vascular complication of diabetes mellitus and a leading cause of poor vision, and blindness globally. Nearly all patients with DMT1 and less than 60% with DMT2 will have some form of diabetic retinopathy (DR) within 20 years of developing diabetes Mellitus while no specific dietary patterns and characteristics have conclusively been shown to reduce DR.

Dietary intake and diabetic retinopathy: A systematic Review: Mark Y. Z. Wong(117) the evidence linking dietary intake with diabetic retinopathy (DR) is growing but unclear. This systematic review between dietary intake and DR showed that dietary fiber, oily fish, and a Mediterranean diet are associated with a lower risk of DR.

Can I Reverse Diabetic Nephropathy and Retinopathy with a Ketogenic Diet? DR Stephen Phinney (118) we have many anecdotes of reversal of neuropathy and nephropathy in people with DMT2 following a well-formulated ketogenic diet but there are no objective data to provide evidence that this is true.

Our observational study shows 5 diabetic patients who had an improvement in DR while treated with LCHF (Ketogenic) diet. There are many anecdotes of reversal of diabetic nephropathy, retinopathy and neuropathy in people with DMT2 following a well-formulated ketogenic diet, they are not published peer-

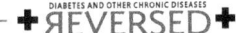

reviewed studies; however, it has been shown that *beta*-hydroxybutyrate, a major ketone produced as a result of ketogenic diet inhibits diabetic retinal damage.

Activation of HCA2 receptors by the beta-Hydroxybutyrate (BHB) inhibits Diabetic Retinal Damage through Reduction of Endoplasmic reticulum Stress and NLRP3 Inflammasome: Trotta M. C. et al (119) while the retinal endoplasmic reticulum markers were elevated in diabetic mice and high NLR3 inflammasome activity, these levels were significantly reduced by the intraperitoneal treatment with BHB. This data suggests that the systematic treatment of diabetic mice with BHB activates retinal HCAs and inhibits local damage. This could offer a therapeutic agent for the treatment of diabetic retinopathy.

Diabetic Gastropathy: A practical approach to a vexing problem: Bo Shen et al (120) although glucose control and dietary changes and drug therapy are current mainstream treatment, "gastric pacing", and a new technique that stimulates gastric motility may give physicians another management tool.

Diabetic gastro paresis/gastropathy (DG) is a common autonomic neuropathy complication of DMT1 and DMT2. Its symptoms are early satiety, postprandial fullness, bloating, abdominal swelling, nausea, vomiting, and retching and delay in gastric emptying. These symptoms are also found with other diabetic complications like cardiovascular disease, hypertension, and retinopathy.

The development of gastro paresis is associated with poor glycemic control. Pharmacological management, glycemic control, nutritional control, and lifestyle modifications are used in the management of DG **(77)**

A LCHF diet assists in glycemic control and subsequent improvement of autonomic function in patients with DG.

KEY TAKEAWAYS:
- *Diabetic nephropathy can be reversed by a simple dietary intervention (LCHF).*

- *It is never too late for a patient to benefit from a LCHF diet.*
- *The improvement of Diabetic Retinopathy by LCHF diet is due to inhibition of retinal damage by the ketone – BHB.*

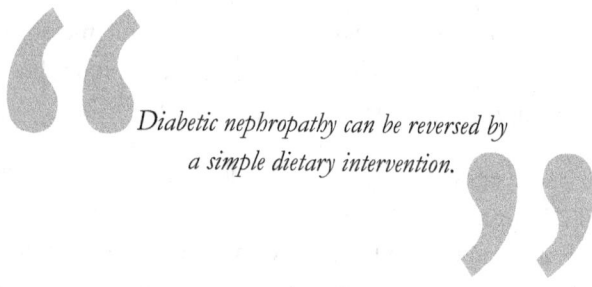

Diabetic nephropathy can be reversed by a simple dietary intervention.

CHAPTER TWENTY FOUR

OTHER APPLICATIONS OF THE LCHF KETOGENIC DIETS

Although it did not feature in our Observational Study; LCHF ketogenic diet has other clinical applications:

1. In the treatment of Polycystic Ovary Syndrome (PCOS).

PCOS is the most common endocrine disorder affecting women of reproductive age and is associated with obesity, hyperinsulinemia and insulin resistance.

*Polycystic Ovary Syndrome, Insulin Resistance, and Inflammation: Brooke Bailey, Stephen Phinney, Jeff Volek: Virta Health; Jan 15, 2019 (121)*Insulin resistance is linked to inflammation and polycystic ovary syndrome (PCOS)leading to chronic pain symptoms and infertility. A well-formulated ketogenic diet and its known effects on Insulin resistance and inflammation can help.

PCOS is associated with abdominal pain, heavy and or irregular menstrual cycles, increased body hair, dark skin patches, mood disturbances, and infertility.

Diagnosis criteria require typically 2 of 3 primary characteristics of
1. Androgen excess (can present as increased body hair).
2. Chronic oligo/ovulation can present as an absent or irregular cycle.
3. The presence of polycystic ovaries at the time of diagnosis.

Underlying all these primary characteristics are two common components of many metabolic diseases; Insulin resistance and inflammation which are also associated with metabolic conditions like diabetes Type-2 (DMT2), obesity, dyslipidemia, and Non-Alcoholic Fatty Liver Disease (NAFLD). Women with PCOS have 2 to 4 times greater chance of developing prediabetes, DMT2, gestational diabetes, obesity, and all these metabolic disturbances increase long term risk of cardiovascular complications and endometrial cancer.

Chronically elevated Insulin signals to the ovary leads to increased androgen production which causes excess abdominal fat gain and the cycle continues.

Insulin resistance in 70% of women with PCOS causes hyperinsulinemia. In PCOS there is Impaired Glucose Tolerance (IGT), a predictor for the development of prediabetes or DMT2. Dietary changes, exercise, and metformin are conventional treatments for PCOS.

All inflammatory markers e.g. WBC, CRP, IL-6 are increased in PCOS. A well-formulated low carbohydrate ketogenic diet (WFKD) reduces all inflammatory markers in addition to reducing Insulin resistance and facilitating weight loss.

Reducing inflammation reduces painful menstrual periods. A WFKD improves the hormonal profile and increases the chance of conception without the use of fertility drugs or medically induced ovulation and their side effects. WFKD also leads to improvement in weight, blood pressure, glucose control and dyslipidemia which are associated with increased cardiovascular disease risk.

*The Effects of a Low Carbohydrate diet on Polycystic Ovary Syndrome: A pilot study Mavropaulos et al (122)*Polycystic Ovary Syndrome is the most common endocrine disorder affecting women of reproductive age and is associated with obesity, hyperinsulinemia, and insulin resistance. Because low carbohydrate diets have been shown to reduce insulin resistance, this pilot study investigated the six month metabolic and endocrine effects of a low carbohydrate ketogenic diet (LCKD) on overweight and obese women with PCOS.

The LCHF ketogenic diet led to significant reductions in weight, percent free testosterone, LH/FSH ratio and Fasting Serum Insulin in women with obesity and PCOS over six months; two women with previous infertility became pregnant

Conclusion:
A LCKD led to significant improvement in weight, percent free testosterone, LH/FSH ratio and fasting insulin in women with obesity and PCOS over 24 weeks.

2. Epilepsy in children.
The ketogenic diet is an established treatment for refractory pediatric epilepsy.

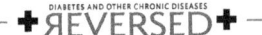

The Ketogenic diet for the treatment of childhood epilepsy: A randomized controlled trial: Neal et al (123) The ketogenic diet has been used widely and successfully to treat children with drug-resistant epilepsy since the 1920s. This study aimed to test the efficacy of the ketogenic diet in a randomized controlled trial.

The results from the trial of the ketogenic diet support its use in children with treatment-resistant epilepsy.

A systematic review of the use of the Ketogenic diet in childhood epilepsy: Keene D. L. et al (124) This was a systematic review of the efficacy, adverse reactions, and costs associated with the diet.

Outcome measures were:
- Degree of seizure control
- Duration patients remained on the diet
- The occurrence of adverse events

The studies indicated that some children report a reduction in seizure frequency. Adverse effects were not frequent; no cost/benefit studies were located.

There is evidence to support the cautious use of the ketogenic diet in refractory epilepsy.

Ketogenic diet and other dietary treatments for epilepsy: Review article: Cochrane Database: Martin k et al (125) The ketogenic diet being high in fat and low in carbohydrates has been suggested to reduce seizure frequency. It is currently used mainly for children who continue to have seizures despite treatment with anti-epileptic drugs. Recently there has been increasing interest in less restrictive ketogenic diets including the Modified Atkins Diet (MAD) and the use of these diets has extended into adult practice.

The objective was to review the efficacy and tolerability of KD and similar diets. Seizure freedom as high as 55% in a 4:1 KD group and seizure reduction of 85% after 3 months were recorded. There were no significant differences in fasting onset and gradual onset KD on seizure freedom.

The MAD reported seizure freedom of up to 10% and seizure reduction of up to 60%. The MAD compared to KD 4:1 did not show a difference in seizure freedom or reductions; adverse effects were consistent in different dietary interventions. Most adverse effects were gastrointestinal syndromes. The randomized trials show promising results for the use of KDs in Epilepsy. **(74).**

3. **Other chronic Neurodegenerative Diseasese.g. Autism, Parkinson's disease, Amyotrophic Lateral Sclerosis, Narcolepsy, Metabolic disorders e.g. Glycogen Storage diseases.**

*Ketogenic diet in Neuromuscular and Neurodegenerative diseases: Antonio Paoli et al: (126)*Ketogenic diets are used in Obesity, Metabolic Syndrome and Diabetes Mellitus. In neurological disorders, the ketogenic diet is recognized as an effective treatment for drug-resistant epilepsy but emerging data suggests it could also be useful in Amyotrophic Lateral Sclerosis (ALS), Alzheimer's and Parkinson's disease and Mitochondropathies. Some common mechanisms can explain the different effects of Ketogenic Diets.

KD leads to the production of ketone bodies (KBs) by the liver. KD stimulates fasting; it might bring improvement in ALS and Mitochondrial disorders, Parkinson's and Alzheimer's Diseases.

There are many KD mechanisms on neurological and neuromuscular diseases including:

    a)   Provision of energy source i.e. ketone bodies
    b)   A decrease in oxidative stress
    c)   Mitochondrial pathway improvements etc.

Thomas Seyfield et al: 2014: Ketone strong: Emerging evidence for a therapeutic role of ketone bodies in neurological and neurodegenerative diseases (127) Chronic and acute inflammation is linked to obesity, Type-2 diabetes, cancer, epilepsy, Alzheimer's and Parkinson's disease, Traumatic Brain Injury and glioma. Diet and lifestyle contribute to these inflammatory diseases.

Calorie restriction (CR) and ketone bodies reduce hyperglycemia, oxidative stress and chronic inflammation. LCHF ketogenic diet (KD) mimics physiological therapeutic fasting and CR. KD and ketones have powerful therapeutic benefits in neurological, and neurodegenerative disease, Traumatic Brain Injury (TBI) and some malignant brain cancers.

Ketogenic diets for Adults with Neurological disorders: MacDonald JW et al: (128) The review highlights the evidence supporting the use of ketogenic diet in a growing number of neurological disorders in adults and mechanics of therapeutic efficacy including neurotransmission, oxidative stress, and neuroinflammation. Clinical evidence supporting ketogenic diet use in the management of adult epilepsy, migraine headache, Motor Neurone Disease, and other neurologic disorders are highlighted and reviewed. Common side effects including gastrointestinal symptoms, weight loss, and transient dyslipidemia are discussed.

4. **Traumatic brain injury (TBI)**: there are indications that in LCHF ketogenic diet ketones may provide an alternative and readily usable energy source for the brain that might reduce its dependence on glucose metabolism which may be impaired following TBI.

Ketogenic diet as a Treatment of Traumatic Brain Injury: A scoping Review: MacDougale et al: (129) Traumatic Brain Injury (TBI) is a leading cause of mortality and morbidity worldwide. The ketogenic diet has been identified as a potential therapy to enhance recovery after TBI. The purpose of the study was to complete a scoping review and synthesize the evidence regarding the KD and its therapeutic effects in TBI. The KD was demonstrated to reduce cerebral edema, apoptosis, improve cerebral metabolism and behavioral outcomes in rodent TBI. Human trials did not establish much evidence for KDs as a treatment for TBI but safety in humans was established.

Nutrition and Traumatic Brain Injury (TBI): Improving Acute and Subacute Health outcomes in Military Personnel: Erdman et al: (130) Traumatic Brain Injury (TBI) is a Major Combat-Related Injury (MCRI) and a major problem among civilians. This is a very comprehensive review in the treatment and resilience against TBI and includes ketogenic diet in the management.

5. **Migraine**

Ketogenic diet in migraine: Rationale, findings, and perspective: Barbanti et al (131) Ketogenic diet is an established treatment for refractory pediatric epilepsy in children and a promising therapy for diverse neurological diseases. Clinical data on KD in migraine obtained from 150 patients suggest that KD may be rapid onset prophylaxis for

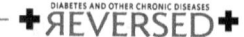
episodic and chronic migraine. KD would contribute to restore brain excitability and metabolism and counteract neuroinflammation in migraines.

6. Non-alcoholic Fatty Liver:

Fatty liver leads to hepatitis, cirrhosis and insulin resistance; it is mainly caused by sugary fructose drinks. Reversing obesity with LCHF diets leads to the reversal of fatty liver.

Fatty Liver and Chemical Pathology: A/Prof Ken Sikaris (132)
Liver functions are:

- a) Synthesize prothrombin time and vitamin K
- b) Excretory: bile salts
- c) Metabolic: lipid, protein, and carbohydrate.

Liver function tests are not direct tests on liver function but are liver damage tests. The liver enzymes are released into plasma when hepatocytes are stressed leading to an increase in AST and ALT. The ratio of ALT/AST determines whether it is a chronic condition or active.

Liver enzymes increase with increase in body weight (AST+ALT). An increase in sugar intake leads to an increase in ALT, cholesterol, and HDL.

Non-alcoholic fatty liver (NAFL) risk factors are Obesity, DMT2,Insulin resistance, dyslipidemia, hypertension **and** polycystic ovary syndrome (PCOS). **Causes of fatty liver**: are fructose e.g. soft drinks cause damage to liver cells and inflammation (hepatitis), leading to fibrosis, and cirrhosis. NAFL leads to Insulin resistance and therefore every organ in the body gets fatty e.g. muscles, heart, and fatty pancreas.

The diagnosis of NAFL is by ALT level or MRI. Obesity leads to fatty liver (NAFL) leading to liver cirrhosis. Weight loss reverses NAFL e.g. LCHF diet. With 10% of total body weight loss NAFL and all markers of metabolic syndrome disappear and it does not matter the method used to lose the weight E.g. Ketogenic diet or Bariatric Surgery

Summary

1. Fatty liver is common. High ALT more than 30 is a sign of Fatty Liver disease.

2. Fatty liver may be the cause of Insulin resistance due to fatty pancreas and fatty muscles
3. Fatty liver is easily reversible by weight loss (10-15%).

LCHF ketogenic diet is an effective way of reversing fatty liver.

7. Sports endurance and performance

Ketogenic diet and endurance: Performance still controversial after four decades: DR Stephen Phinney (133) In1921 Stefanson spent a long time with the Inuits who lived on the Paleo diet.

In the 1880's Arctic explorer explains 'Keto adaptation'; "The weakness after feeding on Reindeer meat passes away in 2-3 weeks".

The 1928 Bellevue Stefanson Experiment: He survived on a very High Fat Diet (more than 80%), medium protein (15-20%) and very low carbohydrate (less than 2%)

In 1930, Study on work performance and nutrition in Germany and Sweden on very high fat low carb diet for few days which showed the low carb diet to be superior.

Keto adaptation was demonstrated:
    a) Vermont study in 1980 using obese patients on a ketogenic diet for 6 weeks.
    b) Keto adaptation confirmed using MIT Bike Racer study which showed much-decreased glycogen quantity and use after keto-adaptation (after 4 weeks) during exercise.

Keto adaptation in trained cyclists was analyzed by Prof Volek which showed a 4-week low carb diet did not compromise endurance performance but was accompanied by adaptation shift from carbohydrates to fat.

How long does it take for humans to adapt? Organic acids and Time Course of Renal Keto Adaptation: Initially uric acid (UA) and *beta*-hydroxybutyrate (BHB) compete for excretion, therefore serum UA rises in the first week and slowly decreases. Renal keto adaptation takes 8 plus weeks to allow normal UA clearance in the presence of continued ketonuria. Therefore a professional sports athlete or in a military environment one needs to be in the low carbohydrate diet for many weeks to achieve full endurance capacity.

In the FASTER Study 2016, two groups on high and low carbohydrate diet were compared; there were more ketones and fat burning (fat oxidation) in the keto adapted group but no difference in glycogen levels.

Endurance even in the military can be enhanced by the ketogenic diet (Tactical Athletes in Nutritional Ketosis (TANK) study. The KD resulted in greater loss of body mass, whole body and visceral fat without calorie restrictions and better performance parameters.

To get good endurance and performance, start KD a long time before or even 2 years before the competition.

Ten (10) reasons why the high capacity to utilize lipid-based fuel benefits Athletes:

1. Fat is stored in greater quantities i.e. 10 times more than carbohydrates.
2. Fat is a more efficient source of fuel than carbohydrates.
3. There is decreased need for fuel during exercises.
4. Ketones reduce oxidative stress.
5. *Beta*-hydroxybutyrate (BHB) signals less inflammation.
6. Enhanced recovery.
7. Keto adapted brain is bonk-proof.
8. Greater ease of weight loss.
9. Augments healthy response to exercise.
10. Enhanced career longevity.

Physical Performance and Ketogenic diets: Prof Volek (134) refers again to the *Faster* Study he did after seeing DR Stephen Phinney's work (Metabolic Characteristics of Keto Adapted Ultra-Endurance Runners). This showed the highest rate of fat oxidation in keto-adapted athletes; higher exercise ketosis, increased LDL and HDL but improved LDL particle distribution (have fewer small LDL particles). KD's use in the military extends the soldier's physical and cognitive performance.

He revisits the TANK study: Which showed that the participants were losing weight but getting stronger with better performance and endurance. *This debunks the long-standing dogma that high carbohydrate intake is required to perform optimally!*

Extended Ketogenic diet and Physical Training Intervention in Military Personnel: Richard A La Fountain et al (135) ketogenic diets elevate ketones into Nutritional Ketosis and are a possible Nutrition approach to address emerging physical readiness and obesity challenge in the Military. This study explored the use of a ketogenic diet in a military population using daily ketone monitoring to personalize the diet prescription.

In conclusion, US military personnel demonstrated high adherence to a KD, improvements in body composition including loss of visceral fat without compromising performance adaptations to exercise training.

Implementation of a Ketogenic diet represents a credible strategy to enhance overall health and readiness of Military Service Members who could benefit from weight loss and improved body composition.

The ketogenic diet has potential even in the military; it's been shown that the obese in the military can lose weight without having to count calories or compromising performance.

8. **Oxygen Toxicity seizures(46).** This is important in deep-sea divers.
9. **Skin diseases** e.g. Acne and psoriasis:

Ketones, ketogenic diet, and the skin: A review of where we are and where we should go: Brianna MacDaniel et al (136) the ketogenic diet has been employed in the prevention and treatment of disease. This article reviews how ketones and Ketogenic diets (KD) can be utilized **in** Dermatology. KD has been used in the treatment of epilepsy, neurodegenerative disease, malignancy, cardiovascular and autoimmune diseases, diabetes, obesity, sports, and combat performance.

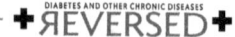
The ketone *beta*-hydroxybutyrate specifically suppresses the activity of the NLRP3 inflammasome which serves as the activating platform for the Interleukin (IL-1B) which is associated with several dermatological diseases (Inflammatory syndromes including Behcet's Disease, Hidradenitis Suppurativa and metastatic melanoma, etc.)

Further studies are needed to ascertain the therapeutic manner the interaction of the NLRP3 inflammasome and IL-1B can be applied/tried on acne, diabetes, diabetic skin diseases, dermatological malignancy and oxidative stress (which is associated with acne, psoriasis, cutaneous malignancy, varicose veins, and drug-induced photosensitivity).

Nutrition and acne: Therapeutic potential for ketogenic diets: Antonio Paoli et al (137)Influence of nutrition on skin health is a growing research area but the findings of various studies on the effect of diet on the development of acne often have been contradictory. This review examines the evidence supporting the influence of various dietary components on the development of acne particularly focusing on the role played by carbohydrates.

The physiological and biochemical effects of the ketogenic diet are examined from this perspective and mechanisms proposed via which this diet could have a role in the treatment of acne.

KEY TAKEAWAYS:

- *The LCHF diet is also used in the treatment of childhood epilepsy, migraine, polycystic ovary disease (PCOS), non-alcoholic fatty liver, oxygen toxicity seisures, chronic neurodegenerative diseases, traumatic brain injury, skin diseases, and it enhances physical performance and endurance.*

CHAPTER TWENTY FIVE

ADVERSE REACTIONS/SIDE EFFECTS OF LCHF KETOGENIC DIETS

There are many listed side effects of LCHF ketogenic diets:

a) **Short term side effects a**re nausea, vomiting, headache, constipation, dehydration, anorexia, lethargy, hypoglycemia, acidosis, and keto rash.

b) **Long term side effects a**re disruption of lipid metabolism, severe hepatic steatosis, hypoproteinemia, mineral deficiencies, increased redox imbalance, cardiomyopathy, and Nephrolithiasis.

In our observational study, the common side effects observed during the LCHF diet therapy inpatient stay were: hypoglycemia, headache, nausea and vomiting, abdominal discomfort, and constipation. All these were mild.

Hypoglycemia required gradual withdrawal of glycemic control agents and headache was treated with additional salt intake.

Are there adequate macro and micronutrients in the ketogenic diets?

There is no standard LCHF diet that suits every patient. A qualified Dietician/Nutritionist should be able to formulate the LCHF diet using locally available, affordable foodstuffs (considering patients' food allergies, etc.) and come up with a macro and micronutrient adequate diet fit for that particular patient.

A definite guide to micronutrients in ketogenic diets is a valuable tool. ***Definite Guide to Micronutrients the Ketogenic Diet: Matt Titlow (138) "Using US Nutritional Institute of Health Recommended intake and the various foodstuffs recommended for KD diet;*** he analyses the micronutrients likely to be lacking (or not lacking) in the American Standard Ketogenic Diet.

DR Loren Cordain: Ketogenic Diets: Long Term Nutritional and Metabolic Deficiencies: (139) This article defines that ketogenic diet has carbohydrate less than 50gm per day using the popular ketogenic diet (KD) common food nutrients and the US dietary recommendations and makes various conclusions on nutrient deficiencies which may occur. There is an obvious bias towards a Paleo diet.

Wajeed Masood: Ketogenic diet March 2019: PubMed: (106)Says" This is a review article on the ketogenic diet (KD), history, ketones, adverse effects, cautions, contra-indications, and clinical significance.

The common minor short term side effects of KD include nausea, vomiting, headache, fatigue, dizziness, difficulty in exercise tolerance and constipation; sometimes referred to as 'Keto Flu', because the KD results in glycogen depletion with its accompanying water and mineral loss. These symptoms resolve in a few days or weeks. Ensuring adequate electrolyte intake counteracts some of these symptoms.

Long term adverse effects of a KD (which are not well formulated) include hepatic steatosis, hypoproteinemia, kidney stones, vitamin and mineral deficiencies in classical KD used in refractory pediatric epilepsy, severe hypoglycemia in diabetic patients on insulin or oral hypoglycemic agents can occur and these medications require adjustments before initiating and during KD.

Other contraindications to KD include pancreatitis, liver failure, and rare metabolic disorders e.g. primary carnitine deficiency, and porphyria.

KEY TAKEAWAYS:

- *The common side effects of the LCHF diet are minor and manageable.*
- *There is no standard LCHF diet that suits every patient. A qualified Dietician/Nutritionist should be able to formulate the LCHF diet using locally available, affordable foodstuffs.*
- *The LCHF diet is Real Food.*
- *The LCHF Ketogenic side-effects, both cognitive and allergic appear fewer than most side effects from medications.*
- *A well formulated LCHF diet has adequate essential macro and micronutrients.*

CHAPTER TWENTY SIX

INFLAMMATION

Inflammation is a natural body immune system response to injury, irritation or infection. Acute inflammation is a healing process. Chronic inflammation is prolonged response where original assault has not been resolved; it involves a progressive change in the type of cells present at the site of inflammation and is associated with simultaneous destruction and repair of the tissue involved.

Factors that induce chronic inflammation are bacterial, viral, parasitic, chemicals, non-digestible particles e.g. asbestos, etc. Inflammatory cytokines if uncontrolled can lead to inflammation.

Inflammation is important in metabolic regulation since unresolved low grade chronic inflammation is a feature of many chronic conditions including metabolic syndrome and cardiovascular disease. Therefore, chronic inflammation leads to various chronic inflammatory diseases e.g. Diabetes Type-2, Atherosclerosis, fibromyalgia, depression, etc.

Non-communicable diseases (NCDs) account for 63% of worldwide deaths. The etiology of these diseases can be traced back to chronic inflammation i.e NCDs like obesity, Diabetes Mellitus, cardiovascular disease, stroke, cancer, chronic respiratory disease, neurological disease e.g. Alzheimer's diseases, autoimmune disease, arthritis and inflammatory bowel disease.

Causes of inflammation include tobacco, alcohol, unhealthy diet (sugar, processed foods, and vegetable oils), visceral obesity, poor sleep, stress, lack of exercise, and lack of sun exposure, etc.

Markers of inflammation are blood cellular markers, soluble mediators, adhesion molecules, adipokines, acute phase proteins e.g. C-reactive protein (CRP), transcription factors and inflammatory enzymes. The markers are non-specific and there is a wide variation in the measurements due to age, diet, body fat, genetics, exercise, etc. and it is not easy to differentiate the ones for low grade,

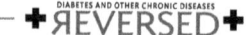
acute or chronic inflammation. The commonly used markers are high sensitive CRP (hs-CRP) and Interleukin-6 (IL-6).

Various foodstuffs affect inflammatory markers differently. The following foods elevate inflammatory markers: high glycemic index carbohydrate foods, lectins, gluten - mainly in wheat and omega 6 fatty acids, etc.

Some foodstuffs that decrease inflammatory markers are: fiber, flavonoids in fruits, and Omega 3 fatty acids.

Dairy products are anti-inflammatory in subjects with metabolic disorders but are inflammatory in subjects allergic to bovine milk **(81)**

Chronic inflammation leads to Low HDL, high LDL particles, high VLDL/triglycerides, high Lipoprotein (a), Insulin Resistance/Hyperinsulinemia, high CRP and Hyperglycemia. All these factors are associated with factors that increase cardiovascular risk e.g. Diabetes, hypertension, obesity, etc.

To reduce chronic inflammation, we have to remove the factors that increase chronic inflammation e.g. stop smoking, and remove inflammatory diet **(84)**. *LCHF diet has massive anti-inflammatory effects.*

A comparison of low fat and low carbohydrate diets on circulating fatty acids and composition and markers of inflammation: Forsythie C E; Stephen Phinney et al (140), abnormal distribution of plasma fatty acids are prominent features of Metabolic Syndrome.

In summary a very low carbohydrate diet resulted in profound alterations in fatty acid composition and reduced inflammation compared to a low fat diet.

The ketones produced by the diet lead to a reduction of fatty acids and inflammatory markers with associated fat loss, increase in glycemic control, Insulin sensitivity and better blood works, specifically triglycerides and HDL which are blood markers for cardiovascular disease. This shows the beneficial non-weight effects of the ketogenic diet.

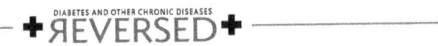

Reduce inflammation: Why Ketogenic diets and exogenous ketones are Key: Brianna Stubbs: PH D (141) explains how ketone bodies especially *beta*-hydroxybutyrate (BHB) affect inflammation.

Inflammation is the body's response to initiate tissue repair; it is linked to infectious and non-infectious diseases e.g. obesity, CVD, DMT2, cancer. Inflammation is acute vs chronic, local or systemic due to inducers, sensors, mediators and target tissue. Inducers are exogenous or endogenous.

Positive effects of ketones on inflammation:

a) **Low-fat v/s low carbohydrate diet on the reduction of inflammation** *(120)*, the keto group lost more weight, the fat mass had low glycemic control, improved insulin sensitivity and better blood work especially triglycerides and HDL, lipoprotein ratios went down, and inflammatory markers decreased in correlation with weight loss.

b) **Anti-inflammatory effects of BHB**; the ketone metabolite BHB blocks NLRP3 inflammasome-mediated inflammatory disease. The inflammasome drives many metabolic diseases due to inflammation e.g. Crohn's disease, DMT2, Alzheimer's disease, atherosclerosis.

c) **BHB protects against eye inflammation**; the activation of retinal HCA2 receptor by systemic BHB inhibits diabetic retinal damage through the reduction of endoplasmic reticulum stress and NLRP3 inflammasome. This shows that BHB protects/reverses diabetic retinopathy. The anti-inflammatory effect of the ketogenic diet is also due to *beta*-hydroxybutyrate (BHB) which directly reduces the inflammation response.

The ketone metabolite beta-hydroxybutyrate blocks NLRP3 inflammasome mediated inflammatory disease: Yourn Y Hee et al (142) **the** ketone bodies Beta-hydroxybutyrate (BHB) and acetoacetate support mammalian survival during states of an energy deficit by serving as an alternative source of ATP. BHB levels are elevated by starvation, caloric restriction, high-intensity exercise, and the low-carbohydrate diet. Prolonged fasting reduces inflammation and BHB reduces inflammatory markers. Therefore, the anti-inflammatory effects of

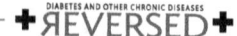
caloric restriction or ketogenic diet may be linked to BHB-mediated inhibition of the NLRP3 Inflammasome.

BHB has also been shown to protect against eye inflammation; therefore reducing diabetic retinopathy.

Activation of HCA2 receptors by the beta Hydroxybutyrate (BHB) inhibits Diabetic Retinal Damage through Reduction of Endoplasmic reticulum Stress and NLRP3 Inflammasome: Trotta M C et al (119) while the retinal endoplasmic reticulum markers were elevated in diabetic mice and high NLR3 inflammasome activity, these levels were significantly reduced by the intraperitoneal treatment with BHB. This data suggests that the systematic treatment of diabetic mice with BHB activates retinal HCAs and inhibits local damage. This could offer a therapeutic agent for the treatment of diabetic retinopathy.

It shows the reduction of chronic inflammation by a ketogenic diet as evident by a reduction in inflammatory markers leads to the reversal of most of the non-communicable diseases (NCDs) which are known to be associated with chronic inflammation.

Ketogenic diet and metabolic therapies: Expanded roles in health and disease: Susan A Masino (143) edited by Susan Masino; this book covers various medical applications of ketogenic diets: treatment of Malignant brain cancer, Alzheimer's disease, traumatic brain, and spinal cord injury, mood disorders, migraine, endocrine disorders, etc. It is a very valuable book for use in broadening knowledge on dietary management of many non-communicable diseases (NCDs)".

Nutrition and inflammation: DR Gary Fettke (144) modern diseases (NCDs) are related to inflammation: DMT1&2, cancer, CVD, dementia, neurological disease, osteoporosis, autoimmune disease, obesity etc. All these diseases are increasing.

Modern medicine focuses on the disease rather than the cause. Nutrition plays a role in inflammation with other factors e.g. stress, cortisol, genetics, chemicals,

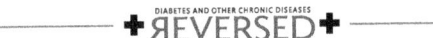
bowel organisms, exercise, latitude/longitude, sleep, vitamin D, and artificial lighting.

The disease model of modern disease: Dietary inflammation is influenced by fructose and other carbohydrates, refined carbohydrates, and polyunsaturated fats. Fructose is changed to uric acid which is used to make nitric oxide which affects blood flow to the brain, increases blood pressure and slows immunity. Fructose causes insulin resistance and it is a leptin inhibitor. This causes an increase in small dense LDL particles. LDL filled with saturated fat has less small oxidized particles while LDL from polyunsaturated fats (PUFs) has more of these particles, therefore it is more Atherogenic.

A high dose of fructose in summer is cleared by vitamin D but in winter, high fructose is not cleared, leading to inflammation.

LDL and cell membranes filled with polyunsaturated fats (PUFs) lead to oxidation, free radicals, inflammation and Atherosclerosis. Dietary carbohydrates have 3% fructose. Endogenous fructose production increases Insulin resistance, hyperglycemia resulting in 10 times increase in conversion of glucose to fructose i.e. 30% conversion of glucose to fructose leading to an increase in inflammation and Atherosclerosis.

Sugar, carbohydrate and PUFs intake lead to more small LDL production, oxidation in cell membranes and LDL small particles. In the USA linoleic acid which is a pro-inflammatory omega 6 in human body fat and breast milk has increased.

Interventions to lower inflammation: Low carbohydrate healthy fat (Ketogenic) diets

In longevity cultures, it is what they don't (not what they eat) and community spirit that explains longevity.

Future eating: Eat real food; be mindful of the whole food chain, low carb, healthy fat, normal protein, minimal polyunsaturated fats.

"Sugar makes you hungry; carbohydrates make you fat, polyunsaturated fats make you inflamed and sick" DR Gary Fettke.

KEY TAKEAWAYS:

- *Chronic inflammation causes most non-communicable diseases.*
- *LCHF diets lower inflammation, <u>prevent</u> and reverse chronic diseases*

> *Eat real food; be mindful of the whole food chain, low carb, healthy fat, normal protein, minimal polyunsaturated fats.*

CHAPTER TWENTY SEVEN

EXERCISE AND INTERMITTENT FASTING

In our diabetic clinic, we emphasize on LCHF dietary intervention and lifestyle changes e.g. stopping smoking, reduction or restriction of alcohol intake, stress management, good sleep, and lifestyle physical activity (LSPA) and intermittent fasting (IF).

Exercise is a structured and planned activity, while LSPA are all physical activities included in daily routines e.g. walking to the workplace.

Exercise and LSPA have beneficial effects

a) On diabetic control/reversal: reduces visceral obesity, improves glucose utilization, decreases glucose production from the liver, decreases the Insulin levels in circulation during exercise, helps achieve good control of blood sugar levels with lower dose of oral hypoglycemic agents or Insulin.

b) Cardiovascular effects: it reduces total cholesterol, LDL, blood pressure levels, and incidence of coronary artery disease; increases HDL and arrhythmic thresholds, and improves cardiovascular function and health.

c) Exercise increases autophagy: Exercise types are:

o General aerobic exercises e.g. walking, cycling, swimming

o Aerobics e.g. dancing

o Strength training e. g. Weight lifting, push-ups, and pull-ups

o Flexibility

The intensity of the exercise can be light, moderate or high. The exercise recommendations should consider the risk of hypoglycemia and diabetic complications in individual patients e.g. non-weight bearing exercises should be promoted in patients with autonomic neuropathy.

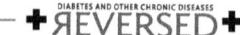
The role of the physician in promoting exercise cannot be overemphasized and a two to four-minute intervention in primary care is enough to promote physical activity.

Patients should be encouraged to have specific, measurable, achievable, realistic and timed goals. Consideration should be given to people with a cardiac history, arthritis, and diabetic complications.

Good hydration, appropriate footwear for peripheral neuropathy and attention to signs and symptoms of hypoglycemia, exercise duration and intensity should be considered. Stress management and seven to eight hours of sleep are recommended.

IDF School of Diabetes: International Diabetes Federation has developed evidence-based educational resources for both diabetes and health professionals and caregivers worldwide (145) which includes exercises for diabetics.

INTERMITTENT FASTING (IF)

Although benefits of IF are many, fasting may result in mild adverse events such as headache, fainting, weakness, dehydration and hunger pangs. Excessive fasting can lead to malnutrition, eating disorders and damage to organs e.g. brain and kidneys. The response to intermittent fasting varies according to gender; women are more sensitive to IF than men. In women, Intermittent Fasting can easily lead to hormonal imbalance which can manifest in menstrual cycle changes.

The risk of hypoglycemia in diabetic patients on oral hypoglycemic agents and or Insulin is common, therefore IF should be done under medical supervision and is generally advisable when patients have been weaned off medications and are on LCHF diet to achieve better glycemic control.

Exercise, calorie restriction and IF increase autophagy: *a process of maintenance of the proteome by balancing synthesis and recycling of intracellular proteins. This process is related to aging and therefore autophagy delays aging and promotes longevity.*

Intermittent fasting has been practiced throughout human history and all major and ancient religions recognize intermittent fasting (IF) to offer physical and spiritual benefits. Although there are many ways of practicing IF, the main purpose is to reduce the duration of eating and increase the fasting duration in a particular period. This can be achieved for example, 24 hour/1day water-only weekly fasting, alternating day water-only fasting, a continuous water-only three-day fasting (although more than three days is not recommended), daily IF e.g. fasting for 16 hours from 8PM to 12noon, 8hours eating window from 12noon to 8Pm: this is the commonest daily IF, and is termed as the 16:8. Some people prefer 18 hours of daily fasting and 6 hour eating window; commonly termed 18:6. Daily IF is easily manageable for people with a regular work schedule.

Diet and nutrition review (146): Moira Lawler has written a lot on health issues: Intermittent fasting has many health benefits:

1. Weight loss as reported in "Nutrition and dietetics 2015"
2. Lowers blood pressure (B/P) "Nutrition and Healthy June 2018"
The 16:8 IF was shown to significantly decrease B/P "Nutrients March 2019"
3. Reduce inflammation "Nutrition Research"
4. Lower cholesterol
A three-week study found lower total cholesterol and LDL cholesterol "Obesity"
5. Boosted Brain function may protect against Brain decline in memory, and amyloid plaques in Alzheimer's Disease "Experimental biology Feb 2018"
6. Cancer protection: Animal studies did show IF can reduce cancer risk by decreasing development of lymphoma, limiting tumor survival and slowing the spread of cancer cells "American journal of cancer prevention"
7. Cell turn over: IF increases autophagy- an important detoxification function in the body to clean out damaged cells. Autophagy creates mTor balance "Autophagy 2018"
8. Reduced insulin resistance (IR): Insulin resistance is a marker of Type-2 Diabetes (DMT2). A study on the therapeutic use of IF for people with DMT2 as an alternative to Insulin showed that 94% of the patients had

decreased medications, 60% had reversed Diabetes and there was a 1-3% average reduction in HbA1c.

Therapeutic use of intermittent fasting for people with diabetes type-2 as an alternative to insulin: Furmli S et al (147) these case series documents three patients referred for Insulin-dependent type-2 diabetes treatment. It demonstrates the effectiveness of therapeutic fasting to reverse Insulin resistance resulting in cessation of their high blood sugars. In addition, these patients were able to lose significant amounts of body weight, reduced their waist circumference and their glycated hemoglobin level (HBA1c).

9. Lower risk of cardiovascular disease due to lower insulin levels.

10. Increased longevity.

Impact of intermittent fasting on health and disease processes: Aging research Reviews: Mattson M P et al (148) Humans in modern societies typically consume food at least three times daily. Overconsumption of food with such eating patterns often leads to metabolic morbidities e.g. Insulin resistance, excessive accumulation of visceral fat, etc. particularly when associated with a sedentary lifestyle.

Intermittent fasting (IF) or periodic fasting (PF) in animal models and humans has demonstrated beneficial effects on health and can counteract disease processes and improve a wide range of age-related disorders including diabetes, CVD, cancers and neurological diseases, e.g. Alzheimer's and Parkinson's disease and stroke.

Intermittent fasting interventions for treatment of overweight and obesity in adults: A systematic Review and Meta analyses: Harris L et al (149) the objective was to examine the effectiveness of intermittent energy restriction in the treatment of overweight and obesity in adults when compared to usual care treatment or no treatment.

Intermittent energy restriction (IER) encompasses dietary approaches including intermittent fasting and fasting for two days per week. Despite the recent

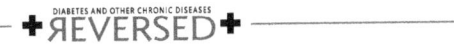
popularity in IER and associated weight-loss claims, supporting evidence base is limited.

The primary outcome of this review was a change in body weight. The conclusion was that IER may be an effective strategy for the treatment of overweight and obesity. IER was comparable to continuous energy restriction for short term weight loss in overweight and obese adults.

Flipping the metabolic switch: Understanding and applying the health benefits of fasting: Anton S D et al (150). Intermittent fasting (IF) is a term used to describe a variety of eating patterns in which no or few calories are consumed for time periods that range from 12 hours to several days on a recurring basis. This review is focused on the physiological responses of major organ systems including the musculoskeletal system. The point of negative energy balance at which liver glycogen stores are depleted and fatty acids mobilized is typically beyond 12 hours after cessation of food intake.

Conclusions: The findings suggest that the metabolic switch from glucose to fatty acids, acid-derived ketones represents an evolutionarily conserved trigger point that shifts metabolism from lipid/cholesterol synthesis and fat storage to mobilization of fat through fatty acid oxidation and fatty acid-derived ketones, which serve to preserve muscle mass and function.

Thus intermittent fasting regimens that induce the metabolic switch have the potential to improve body composition in overweight individuals. IF regimens also induce coordinated activation of signaling pathways that optimize physiological function, enhance performance and slow aging and disease processes.

Horne B D et al: *Health benefits of intermittent fasting: Hormesis or Harm: A systematic Review:* (151) Intermittent fasting, alternate-day fasting and other forms of periodic caloric resistance are gaining popularity but it is unclear whether clinical evidence is strong enough to support the use of such dietary regimens as health interventions. Improvements in weight and other related outcomes were found in 3 trials and 2 observational trials showed fasting was associated with lower prevalence of coronary arterial disease and diabetes.

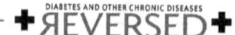
DR Robert Szabo: *Introduction to therapeutic fasting*: **(152)** was diagnosed at 37 years with DMT2 and started current oral diabetes treatment. He stopped metformin and high carbohydrate diet and his sugars stabilized. Intermittent fasting further helped him reverse his DMT2.

History of fasting: Fasting has been practiced through the ages, e.g. Jesus fasted. Fasting has been used for physical and spiritual cleansing.

The Dietary Recommendations encourage eating of many frequent small meals; eat regular meals, don't skip meals and always start the day with breakfast and snack suggestions.

Insulin is a pulseable hormone and frequent meals and snacking leads to Insulin spikes and accompanying stimulation of fat formation. 8 hours of fasting lead to reduced Insulin and fat loss.

Snacking obese people have higher Insulin levels and more Insulin spikes and high leptin blockage. High carbohydrate diet, high fructose diet, and snacks lead to Insulin resistance which is associated with obesity, DMT2, NAFL, dyslipidemia, PCOS, gout, Atherosclerosis, inflammation, hypertension and maybe GERD, Autoimmune diseases, IBS, Alzheimer's and Parkinson's disease, arthritis/allergy, cancers, and Osteopathy.

Insulin resistance is perpetuated by high Insulin and vice versa; a low carbohydrate diet reduces Insulin level and Insulin resistance.

Fasting reduces Insulin resistance as evidenced by a study done on: *Effects of Ramadhan fasting on glucose and homeostasis and adiponectin levels: Gnanou J V et al (153).*

Physiological stages of fasting are: meal, feeding, gluconeogenesis, ketosis i.e. 6 hours post-meal is when fasting starts. Getting started on intermittent fasting:
  i)   More than 6 hours without food
  ii) Up to 5 days with minimum risk
  iii) Start short e.g. 12 hours and gradually extend

DIABETES AND OTHER CHRONIC DISEASES

iv) Experiment and mix it up (16/8), 24hours per week, alternate, multiple-day/combinations
v) Mini fasts; eat only 1 to 2 meals per day.
vi) Drink 3 litres of clear fluids; water, broth, tea, coffee, etc. To supplement sodium, take bone broth, salt, exercise, and work.

Common side effects of intermittent fasting are:

- Hunger up to 3 days
- Agitation due to adrenaline
- Light-headedness
- Diarrhea

But with adrenaline people notice increased focus and efficiency.

Precautions: who should not fast?

- Pregnant women
- Children
- People with a BMI less than 20.
- If you have any medical condition, don't fast without medical supervision.

Potential complications of fasting:

1. Dehydration
2. Electrolyte imbalance (low sodium)
3. Fluid overload (heart failure)
4. Hypoglycemia (hypoglycemic drugs, insulin)
5. Refeeding syndrome (complex, possibly fatal, hypophosphatemia, fasting more than 5 days in non-obese. *Refeeding syndrome: Mehanna (154)*

Summary:

1. Fasting has always been part of human experience; our bodies need it to function optimally.
2. Insulin resistance is the basic reason for most of our modern diseases.
3. Insulin resistance is a dietary disease and therefore curable through dietary manipulation.

4. Fasting is the quickest means of reversing Insulin resistance.

DR Jason Fung and Jimmy Moore: Why you shouldn't fear fasting: Interview: (155) Fasting has benefits beyond weight loss; even stem cell regeneration. The fear of fasting is not justified and the starvation mode is a myth. Fasting is an ancient practice; Buddha, Jesus fasted.

Fasting activates some human hormones; adrenaline, growth hormone, cortisol leading to more energy and rebuilding. It activates autophagy, promotes longevity, anti-aging and anticancer, reverses Alzheimer's disease and DMT2, enhances weight loss and athletic performance-enhancing (train harder and recover faster).

Starvation mode: that when you fast your metabolism slows down and you lose muscle mass is NOT true! During fasting, the body switches on other fuel sources; ketones to maintain an even higher metabolism. Intermittent fasting results in 4 times better preservation of muscle mass than calorie reduction. Ghrelin goes down from day 2 and hunger subsides.

During fasting, milk, bulletproof coffee, bone broth, artificial sweeteners are not advised. Some patients regain more weight after stopping a low-calorie diet than they previously had. Insulin resistance; fasting blood sugar/glucose or insulin levels decrease with intermittent fasting, muscle mass increases as shown by a 'Dexa Scan".

During intermittent fasting persistent low levels of insulin decrease Insulin resistance making it easier to lose weight. HbA1c can be improved by a change in exercise type e.g. bone bending. The reduction of skin tags due to weight loss responds to intermittent fasting due to autophagy.

Women's response to IF is not very different from men. IF is not advised during pregnancy or in patients with low BMI and in children.

Women have been doing religious fasts without any hormonal problems and clinically there are no significant hormonal problems.

IF is easier when one is on KD diets; fasting saves money, time and doesn't affect the thyroid hormone. It is advisable to consider diet, fasting, spiritual and community support.

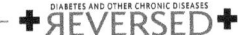

Branthorst S; Longo V D: Dietary restrictions and nutrition in the prevention and treatment of cardiovascular disease (156) Insulin resistance induces hyperglycemia and dyslipidemia and these increase plasma triglycerides, LDL and decreased HDL levels. This trend leads to endothelial dysfunction and the formation of atherosclerotic plaque. Intermittent, periodic fasting and the ketogenic diet have the potential to prevent and treat CVD.

Eschober et al: *Autophagy and aging: Maintaining the proteome through exercise and caloric restriction:* (157) Accumulation of dysfunctional and damaged cellular proteins and organelles occurs during aging. Autophagy is an evolutionary conserved recycling of pathways responsible for the degradation and turnover of cellular proteins and organelles which is linked to aging.

Exercise promotes healthy aging and mitigates age-related pathologies. Caloric restriction (CR) promotes lifespan by augmenting intracellular protein quality. Therefore longevity effects of exercise and CR may stem from the recycling of intracellular proteins and present practical means of promoting longevity.

This article discusses autophagy-mediated effects, mTor and aging, caloric restriction promotes lifespan and health in aging, exercise may maintain the proteome, the role of exercise intensity in the autophagic response, chronic effects of exercise and autophagic activity.

Conclusion
Autophagy and Caloric Restriction positively impacts lifespan and enhances longevity by maintaining the proteome and organelle population.

KEY TAKEAWAYS:

- *Exercise, intermittent fasting and LCHF diet activate autophagy and they also reverse diabetes type-2*
- *Autophagy delays aging and promotes longevity*

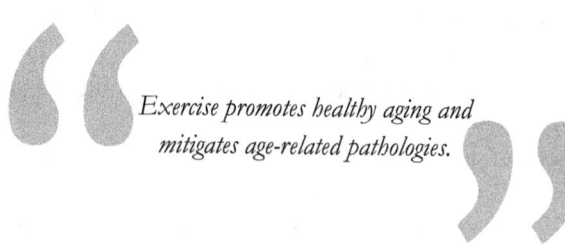

*Exercise promotes healthy aging and
mitigates age-related pathologies.*

CHAPTER TWENTY EIGHT

LCHF DIET (KETOGENIC) AND CARDIOVASCULAR HEALTH

Cardiovascular risk factors include: -

A. Conventional risk factors are age, family history, and race.

B. Modifiable risk factors are high blood cholesterol levels especially Low-Density Lipoproteins (LDL), high blood pressure, cigarette smoking, diabetes Mellitus, obesity, lack of physical activity, Metabolic syndrome, mental stress, and depression.

C. Non-traditional or novel risk factors are high C-Reactive protein (CRP), lipoprotein (a)

Homocysteine, small dense LDL-C particles, and fibrinogen

D. Advanced renal disease, HIV

To measure patient's progress and cardiovascular risk, the following should be looked at: LDL, High-density lipoprotein (HDL), Total cholesterol (TC): HDL, Triglyceride (TG): HDL ratios

In interpreting lipid profile, look at the whole picture; TC: HDL Ratio, TG: HDL Ratio, Specifics of LDL: LDL-P, ApoB, size density, and oxidation. Put in context with metabolic Health:

- Insulin or Insulin resistance (IR) HbA1c, (OGTT) Oral glucose Tolerance Test

- Inflammation (CRP)

- Blood Pressure (B/P), visceral adipose metabolic health

- The Coronary Calcium score is gaining importance as a reliable marker of cardiovascular risk and so is Carotid Intima-Media Thickness (CIMT).

However, recent trials have shown that dietary saturated fats do not lead to increased cholesterol and there is no relationship between high cholesterol and heart disease:

1. There is no significant prolongation of life span due to statins use, considering their side effects.
2. Saturated fats are not associated with cardiovascular disease.
3. Cardiovascular disease is multifactorial.
   LDL physiological role and glycated LDL as a marker of cardiovascular risk need to be reviewed carefully; in vascular injury and plaque rupture, the risk factors are mainly insulin resistance, inflammation, oxidation, and endothelial dysfunction.
4. Cardiovascular risk can be lowered without LDL reduction e.g. Stop smoking, reverse diabetes and improve lifestyle e.g. physical activity, sleep, stress management, and social connections.

LCHF (ketogenic) diet has the following benefits:

a) Increased (HDL) Lowered Triglycerides (TG)
b) Improved insulin sensitivity and glucose control
c) Treatment and reversal of Diabetes
d) Reversal of metabolic syndrome
e) Weight loss, specifically fat loss
f) Decreased inflammation
g) Improved energy
h) Decreased hunger:**(17) (18) (19)(20)(23) (27)(28)(29)(55)(111)**

DR Paul Mason: *High cholesterol on a ketogenic diet (plus do statins work)? 2019 uptake: (158)* LDL is said to be BAD and that's why statins are a BIG SALE. There is a *lack of an association or an inverse association between low-density lipoprotein - cholesterol and mortality in the elderly* systematic review *(159)*

16 of these reviews found an inverse relationship between LDL and All-cause mortality; the higher the LDL, the lower All-cause mortality.

Medical insurance application can fail due to high cholesterol and LDL but cholesterol and LDL are essential for good health. LDL can be good or bad.

Complex carbohydrates cause high blood sugar and "damaged" LDL. Cholesterol refers to chylomicron, VLDL, IDL, and LDL depending on their size and HDL all are lipoproteins; then they are recycled back to the liver.

LDL is released from the liver, they carry fat into tissues and release ApoA and ApoB.

Sugar from carbohydrates makes the LDL receptors in the liver NOT to recognize LDL particles leading to small dense LDL; glycated or oxidized LDL. Therefore these particles cannot be taken up by the liver and end up in the blood in peripheral tissues and accumulate i.e. increase in small LDL particles which is a better predictor of CVD risk. Small LDL particles enter the vessel wall lining (glycocalyx) which is damaged by high circulating blood sugar and leptin. Oxidized LDL leads to atherosclerosis or narrowing of coronary arteries.

Oxidized LDL can be analyzed by centrifugation or antibodies of the oxidized LDL. Lipoprotein Apo A is related to CVD risk.

Statins increase liver receptors for LDL but NOT oxidized LDL. Therefore the ratio of oxidized LDL to non-oxidized LDL increases. Statins lead to an average increase in lifespan by 5.2 days if you have a history of cardiovascular disease and if no history of CVD by 3.1 days.

Side effects of statins:
1 in 10 patients could not tolerate any statin due to severe rhabdomyogia/muscle pains, 1 in 5 could not tolerate due side effects of maximum dose.

Therefore a patient who has high cholesterol and high LDL is healthy and fit for medical insurance.

DR S Phinney and DR Mackenzie: *How does VIRTA affect heart health and cardiovascular risk?*(160) All18 cardiovascular risk factors were decreased but LDL initially rises although the smaller dense LDL which are atherogenic and recognized to be related to high CVD risk decrease. HDL cholesterol/triglycerides ratio increases but hypertension leading to de-prescription of medication, inflammation, hs-CRP, and WBC decreased.

*DR Sarah Hallberg MD: Ketogenic diet and heart disease: New research updates: (161)*she expresses her frustration with Conventional diabetes and obesity treatment and then switched to low carbohydrate high-fat diet and noted impressive results. As an Obesity Specialist, obesity and diabetes treatment include low carb without/with caloric restriction and or medications.

Conventional DMT2treatment leads to more medications but the elimination of carbohydrates reverses diabetes. The gradual removal of diabetes medications should be supervised to prevent hypoglycemic events on the introduction of a low carb diet.

Summary:
1. When DR Hallberg opened a low carb Clinic, they quickly saw weight loss and reversal of Diabetes.
2. Hallberg is part of the largest and longest trial of Nutritional Ketosis as a treatment to reverse diabetes type-2.
3. Exercise and low carb/Keto are now considered as treatment options for obesity.
4. Medications are used for treatment of diabetes symptoms but not for the progression of the disease, each step in medication speeds up the cycle.
5. Continuous glucose monitors allow you and your doctor to know blood sugar levels between finger pricks.
6. Remote care/telemedicine
7. Most Americans have some sort of metabolic issue; over 50% of adults have diabetes or prediabetes.
8. With Nutritional Ketosis you can reverse diabetes and improve cardiovascular risk factors e.g. a significant decrease in blood pressure and triglycerides, and a significant increase in good cholesterol/HDL.
9. A better cardiovascular risk marker than LDL is LDL-P for type-2 diabetes or those with insulin resistance.
10. Inflammatory markers especially C-reactive protein (CRP) decreased by 40% over the study year.
11. It is best to consume 3-5 grams of Sodium a day.
12. Biomarkers: Blood pressure, blood sugar, HDL Cholesterol, decrease in triglycerides, LDL cholesterol small particles, CRP, weight, and blood ketones.

13. Serum ketone goals are above 0.5mmol of *beta*-hydroxybutyrate (BHB). There may be a role for ketosis even at lower levels.

14. Diabetes medications lower blood sugar acutely but cardiovascular outcomes were NOT improved. With SGLT-2 inhibitors, there was improvement with cardiovascular mortality.

15. SGLT-2 inhibitors inhibit reabsorption of glucose and can lead to dangerously high levels of ketones.

16. Metformin affects gut hormones and the microbiome.

17. The American Diabetes Association (ADA) guidelines are not evidence-based.

18. DASH diet, recommended by ADA can make diabetes worse.

19. We need to change the dietary guidelines as they impact all of us.

20. For proper meta-analyses, you need to pay attention to the inclusion criteria.

Kosinski et al: Effects of ketogenic diets on cardiovascular risk factors: Evidence from animal and human studies: (162) Treatment of obesity and cardiovascular disease includes weight loss on Ketogenic diets and their impact on cardiovascular risk factors improvements in obesity and DMT2 have been described.

KD has been associated with a significant reduction in total cholesterol, an increase in HDL cholesterol, a decrease in triglycerides and a reduction in LDL cholesterol levels. KD led to weight loss in humans, could improve Non-Alcoholic Fatty Liver (NAFL), decrease in insulin resistance and DMT2, improvement in lipid profile and reduction in blood pressure.

Uffer Ravnskov et al: LDL-C does not cause cardiovascular disease: A comprehensive review of current literature: (163) For half a century, a high cholesterol or total cholesterol (TC) or low-density lipoprotein cholesterol (LDL-C) has been considered to be the major cause of Atherosclerosis and cardiovascular disease (CVD) and Statin treatment has been widely promoted for cardiovascular prevention. However, there is increasing understanding that the mechanisms are more complicated and that Statin treatment in particular, when used as primary prevention, is of doubtful benefit.

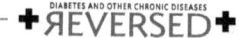

The authors of three large reviews published by Statin advocates have attempted to validate the current dogma. This article delineates the serious errors in these three reviews as well as other obvious falsifications of the Cholesterol Hypothesis.

Expert Commentary:
"Our search for falsifications of the cholesterol hypothesis confirms that it is unable to satisfy any of the Bradford Hill criteria for causality and that the conclusions of the authors of the three reviews are based on misleading statistics, exclusion of unsuccessful trials and by ignoring numerous contradictory observations".

Low carb/high fat and heart: DR Bret Scher: Cardiologist (164) CVD is a major killer but 50-80% of heart attacks are preventable. The 1977 American guidelines failed to prevent the majority of chronic non-communicable diseases. Drugs don't fix the problem. The advice: Eat less, exercise more, and reduce fat does not work and patients are getting heart attacks.

Benefits of LCHF lifestyle: reduce hunger, reduce blood sugar swings, better weight loss, reverse DMT2, and metabolic syndrome, and lower blood pressure.

Other potential benefits: treat and prevent Alzheimer's disease, certain cancers, treat mental disorders and reduce CVD risk.

What about that fat?

Epidemiological studies, randomized trials, and surrogate markers VS clinical endpoints:

Evidence against saturated fat started with Ancel Keys' Fat Heart Hypothesis.

Clinical evidence does not show a relationship between cardiovascular mortality and dietary saturated fats. Saturated fats are not associated with all-cause mortality, CVD, CHD, ischemic stroke or DMT2. In Vegetarians and Vegans, the quality of evidence does not qualify the conclusions.

In the 'blue zones' where people have very high longevity there is more in the way they live than the diet only. They have some commonalities

.**Surrogate markers that back the recommendation for LCHF diet**: lipids, glucose, insulin, blood pressure, inflammatory markers, hip-waist ratio (Butt: gut ratio); others endothelial: CAC, CIMT

1. Lipids: look at the entire profile, not just LDL, HDL, TG-size/density all improve

LCHF v/s low fat diets.

All lipid profiles improve with LCHF diets than low-fat diets even Apo A and Apo B

Framingham Heart Study: LDL alone is not a marker, raising HDL with diet is most effective than with medications. LDL is not the major risk factor in heart attacks.

In people, over 60 years there is a benefit to elevated LDL in terms of longevity and dementia. Lipid ratios are better predictors for CHD risk; they are markers of metabolic health.

JUPITOR TRIAL: LDL reduction in context: There are no LDL/statins studies done on LCHF subjects.

2. LCHF increases HDL, decreases TG and improves LDL particle size, glucose, insulin, reverses metabolic syndrome/insulin resistance, not just diabetes but insulin resistance and diabetes improves too and eliminates medications. Treating diabetes to HbA1c of 7.0 with drugs while maintaining hyperinsulinemia does not decrease cardiovascular risk outcomes but a reduction of HbA1c below 7.0 with accompanying Insulin reduction with lifestyle/diet reduces cardiovascular risk markers.

3. Blood pressure, which is an important cardiovascular risk factor, is easy to measure and improve on the LCHF diet. Salt restriction only helps in 25% of the general patient and is not recommended for the majority of the people. LCHF improves blood pressure more than a low-fat diet plus weight loss drugs (orlistat).

4. Inflammatory markers: is easy to improve from Standard American Diet (SAD). LCHF leads to the consistent improvement of inflammatory markers: the LCHF diet reduces inflammation.

5. Hip-waist (Butt: Gut) ratio; LCHF reduces visceral and body fat.

6. Other markers: Endothelial function e.g. Coronary Calcium score (CAC) and CIMT

CAC score is an important cardiovascular risk factor marker. There is no statin benefit for patients with CAC of 0.

A/Prof Sikaris: HbA1c/Insulin and cardiovascular risk: (165)
Outline:
1. What is HbA1c and diabetes?
2. HbA1c correlation with Diabetes
3. HbA1c correlation with insulin

HbA1c and risk: Albuminuria is an important diabetes risk factor. Lipids, urate, fatty liver, testosterone, and troponin are important Prediabetes and CVD risk factors.

HbA1c is glycated hemoglobin A. It is related to fasting blood glucose levels and is used in the diagnosis of diabetes and its complications e.g. retinopathy, neuropathy. In prediabetes or Metabolic Syndrome HbA1c is 5.7-6.4. The higher the HbA1c, the higher the fasting Insulin. Insulin is broken down into C- Peptide. HbA1c is related to insulin, fatty liver, triglycerides, HDL and CVD risk.

Summary:
HbA1c is a better measure of dysglycemia than glucose. It is a consistent measurement and preferred test for diabetes. It correlates well with albuminuria with time and should be a preferred test for prediabetes.

Prediabetic HbA1c associates with hyperinsulinemia, dyslipidemia, and fatty liver and cardiac damage in time.

*Blood tests to assess your cardiovascular risk: A/Prof Ken Sikaris (166)*LCHF
blood tests for CVD risk are:
a) Blood tests for carbs/Glucose: HbA1c
b) Blood tests for fats: triglycerides, small dense LDL, HDL-c
c) Blood test for other markers: ALT (fatty liver), Urate, and Troponin.

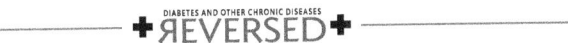

Metabolic syndrome increases CVD risk.

Fasting and random glucose

Fasting glucose: Overnight fast depletes glycogen, glucose levels are dependent on hormones rather than on the size of the meal.

Random glucose: depends on the amount of glucose in a meal and glucose taken up by tissues i.e. Insulin resistance and amount of muscle. Glucose levels vary; therefore HbA1c is more reliable. HbA1c is used to diagnose diabetes and predict diabetic complications.

Small dense LDL correlates with all metabolic syndrome CVD risk factors; triglycerides are important.

Interpretation of blood tests (lipid profiles) and the importance of the following parameters has changed over time:
30 years ago: High cholesterol
20 years ago: Bad cholesterol (LDL-C) and good cholesterol (HDL-C)
10 years ago: Modified LDL Atherogenic, oxidized, glycated, Apo A/Lipoprotein A, small dense LDL
Today: Triglycerides are important.

LCHF diets lead to slightly higher LDL, HDL-c, and TC increase, TC/HDL-c and triglyceride/HDL-c decrease.

Fatty liver correlates with higher triglycerides and low HDL-c, high ALT, GTT, and fasting insulin. Urate which is increased by fructose drinks is a predictor of Metabolic Syndrome. Troponin-T is a marker of heart damage.

Other CVD risk markers are Urine albumin, hs-CRP and homocysteine **(36).**
DR Eric Thorne: Cardiologist: Is keto bad for your heart? (167) Coronary heart disease is a major killer. **Formation of Coronary Vessel plaque and predisposing risk factors:** Saturated fats do not predict CVD risk. Insulin and Insulin resistance is associated with Metabolic Syndrome. Ketogenic diet is a low carbohydrate diet and it lowers Insulin. *Carbohydrate restriction is the most*

effective dietary treatment of obesity and it improves all manifestations of Metabolic Syndrome; weight loss, blood pressure, HbA1c, glucose, total cholesterol (TC), HDL and Triglycerides.

Carbohydrate restriction improves blood pressure irrespective of weight loss and reverses non-alcoholic fatty liver disease. Ketogenic diets reduce inflammation, hs-CRP and has the greatest effect on blood sugar, HbA1c and improves atherogenic dyslipidemia. TC does not change much, HDL increases, triglycerides decrease, LDL may increase slightly but LDL small dense particles decrease.

In a 2018 two-year ketogenic diet patient follow up, all these CVD risk factors were reduced including reduction/discontinuation of blood pressure and diabetic medications: *Is there evidence that ketogenic diet is harmful?* There is no evidence based on all CVD calculators. The ketogenic diet has a 98% risk reduction and it reduces Carotid Artery plaques as much as other diets.

Some studies should be ignored e.g. the recent study that showed low carbohydrate is associated with high mortality. It was based on questionnaires, was NOT randomized, etc. The majority of self-reports of energy intake are incompatible with life! Are other factors considered e.g. sleep, smoking, exercise?

Conclusion:
Low carbohydrate diets are safe and sustainable. There is no 'essential' carbohydrate. Low carbohydrates allow for a wide variety of vegetable intake. Processed foods are reduced on the LCHF diet.
A low carbohydrate diet is not a 'FAD' diet".

KEY TAKEAWAYS:

- *The LCHF diet is heart-healthy. It improves all cardiovascular risk markers e.g. obesity, blood pressure, Insulin, HbA1c, lipid profile, CAC, inflammatory markers (CRP, etc).*
- *Some patients on LCHF have increased LDL, but the LDL small particles which cause heart disease decrease.*

CHAPTER TWENTY NINE

CHALLENGES IN IMPLEMENTING/SUSTAINING LCHF KETOGENIC DIETS

The implementation and sustainability of the LCHF diet starts with recognizing LCHF as a lifestyle and not a diet. The compliance/non-compliance to the LCHF diets is as frequent as with medications for chronic diseases **(168)**. Physicians perceive poor patient motivation as a major reason for non-compliance, although there are many challenges experienced by the patient.

A. General

a) Preconceived beliefs and misinformation on lifestyle diseases e.g. obesity is hereditary, unavoidable, part of normal aging process, medication is a solution or all cure; food is not medicine, LCHF diet is a fad, non-evidence based dietary guidelines e.g. 2hours eating, starvation mode, carbs are essential, promotion of processed foods; eating processed foods is a sign of wealth, distorted definition of healthy food, health associations sponsored by food industry that put out wrong advice e.g. saturated fat and cholesterol kills, vegetable oils are manufactured from vegetables and are cholesterol-free and good for the heart.

b) Food environment: cheap fast food outlets, junk food in supermarkets, billboards, TV adverts, hospital food.

c) New norm: obesity is normal and a measure of "Health"

d) Government and health insurance firms not aware or convinced of the role of LCHF diets in the prevention/treatment of non-communicable diseases.

B. Cultural and religious beliefs.

a) Religious beliefs and festivals with certain high carbohydrate foods which have to be eaten. The notion that only eating certain foods can bring satiety/have nutritional value.

b) Fear of stigmatization.

c)   Obesity is a sign of prosperity; being thin/slim is associated with poverty and disease;

d)   Changed eating culture, traditional foods are for the lower class in the society, and the notion that chronic diseases like diabetes Type-2 are irreversible.

C.   Family
a)   Expectation of disease.
b)   Extended family living.
a)   Lack of support in the family unit.

D.   Individual
a)   Previous medical misinformation e.g. medical, nutritional information by medical personnel.
b)   Denial
c)   Depression
d)   Level of education
e)   Food addiction
f)   Workplace
g)   Time challenge
h)   Secondary gain from being sick

E.   Financial, availability, affordability, and methods of preparing the food.

G.   Common meals especially in schools, colleges, universities, hospitals, military or on travel, lack of Keto restaurants.

H.   Unavailability of local LCHF diet recipes

To overcome these challenges:

a)   The government and Medical training Institutions should amend the current guidelines and policies on the management of Non-communicable Diseases and include LCHF diet option in the Health/Nutrition Curricula.

b) Insurance companies should include the LCHF diet as part of their accepted mode of treatment for non-communicable diseases for their clients.

c) Educate and train patients and medical personnel on LCHF.

d) Learn the patient's lifestyles, habits, and cultural beliefs.

e) Identify stumbling blocks, engage patients in decision making

f) Have practical goals

g) LCHF diet encourages the consumption of meat and meat products. This could be a challenge to Vegans and Vegetarians but LCHF diets to suit these groups are available.

*Efficacy of a moderately Low carbohydrate Diet in a 36-month observational study for Japanese patients with type-2 Diabetes: Mariko Sanada et al (169)*A team of Japanese researchers in a new study set out to find out whether eating a moderate carbohydrate diet is sustainable, effective and safe long term. After 3 years 200 DMT2 patients on moderate carbohydrate restriction (70-130gms) per day was enough to have a positive effect on the patient's health markers' and the diet is highly effective, safe and sustainable".

*Keto sustainability: Carole Freeman: Nutritionist (170)*Diets don't work; they did not work for her. She came across the ketogenic diet, was initially skeptical about it but she lost weight, signs of post-traumatic hypopituitarism and chronic pain disappeared. There are several reasons why people struggle and cheat on the LCHF diet:

a) Neuro-regulation: cravings are a dopamine conditional-response which can be minimized by food cues, TV ads, work environment. There should be no sweets/sweeteners of any kind and people should consume adequate protein.

b) Salt: consume adequate salt, 2.5-4gm of Sodium daily or 1-3 added teaspoon of salt per day. We are wired to eat. What triggers eating or overeating; sensory cues, seeing, Pavlovian conditioning, liquid calories, high palatable foods, variety, and dessert.

c) Strategies to moderate appetite:

- Avoid seeing food, recipes, TV shows, grocery, work environment, no nuts, and seeds with high-carb content.

- Eat food at the right time and do not over-eat
- Avoid liquid fats except for olive oil and liquid calories,
- Eat real food
- Keep meals real simple and do not snack
- Habit loops changing: make keto easier than alternative
- Stress management, e.g. yoga, creates a new habit, social connections.
    a) Make healthy foods affordable
    b) The LCHF diet is sustainable and should not be viewed as only applicable for a short time; it's a lifestyle.

Ruminant reality: Getting to the meat sustainability: Peter Ballerstedt: KETOCON 2018 (171) A Foliage Extension Specialist talks about true social, economic and ecological sustainability of the LCHF diet, ruminant animal production systems, the source of butter, red meat and cheeses!

To those restoring their mental and physical health with a diet containing animal source foods "Don't listen to the voice that sold you the diet that made you sick in the first place! Meat does not make you fat, clog your arteries, cause diabetes, cancer, kill your kidneys, acidify your blood, melt your bones, make you morally weak, deprive you of food or drive climate change.

Ruminant Agriculture is truly sustainable Agriculture which applies the nitrogen fixation cycle. Most of the global protein supply is from animal sources. Protein intake guidelines should not be on a percent of calorie basis and intake should be a specific amount of high-quality protein-based upon individual considerations. Crude estimates overestimate the protein content of foods from plants. The biological value of proteins from animals is 1.4 times that of foods from plants.

Cattle contribute directly to global security because cattle rely on grazing and forages, they need only 0.6kg of protein from human edible feed to produce 1kg of protein in milk and meat, which is of higher nutritional quality than the plant proteins.

A big proportion of the earth is fit for animal agriculture but not suitable for legumes. There is only a quarter of the earth suitable for plant food. Ruminants play an essential role in human nutrition. Ruminant agriculture is the best way of reducing soil erosion and *it does not contribute to significant global warming.*

In the USA all agriculture produces 9% of greenhouse gas emissions (GHG), livestock agriculture produces 4% of GHG, the beef industry produces 2% of GHG emissions and transport produces 28% of US GHG emissions. If we stop all animal agriculture it will reduce GHG by 2.6% in the US and 0.36 globally but it will produce an unbalanced food ecosystem and create essential dietary nutrient deficiencies.

LCHF Challenges: Nicole Moore: Australian Low Carb Dietician (172) discusses the following:
1. Vegan diet in insulin resistance overweight patients
2. Abdominal effects of the LCHF diet
3. Not losing weight on LCHF diet

Macronutrients for LCHF diet: 60% TE fat: 30% TE proteins: 10% TE carbohydrate but theLCHF diet should be individualized to the culture and comorbidities.

Vegan LCHF weight Loss: In the Vegan diet pyramid you have to change macronutrient profile from 10% fat, 30-40% protein, 60% carbohydrate to LCHF 60% fat:30% protein: 10% carbs

Vegan LCHF macronutrient targets
For example in a 1500 calorie weight loss plan:
Target 1500 Calories
a) Fat: 60% 900 calories, 9 calories per gram fat (Atwater Factor) 100gm fat per day but try not to count calories

b) Protein in 1500 calories loss plan
Target calories 1500
Protein 30% calories; 450 calories
4 calories 1gm protein per day (Atwater factor)
113gm protein per day

c) Carbs in 1500 calorie weight loss plan
Target calories 1500
Carbs 10% calories; 150 calories
4 calories/gram carb (Atwater factor) 38gm per day

Maintain RDI (iron/protein)
RDI iron (mg/day) is 8mg/day adults and women (29-50years) 10mg/day

Dropping carbs means: Consume fewer legumes, lentils, soybeans, tofu, linia beans and fewer grains: quinoa, fortified cereals, brown rice, and oatmeal. Legumes/grains are the main sources of iron and proteins.

Vegan LCHF challenges:
They rely on high carb: only vegetable products, legumes, grains, fruit and vegetables (starchy), the battle is to keep carbohydrate intake low; 10% TE.

To get enough protein and iron, vegans eat lots of legumes, grains which are high in protein and iron but they are high in carbohydrates.

a) Low-fat vegan diet: Increased fat sources to 60% meet RDI iron (18mg/day).

Eat more avocado, nuts, coconut olive, and macadamia oil.

b) Low carb vegan protein

Coconut milk, yogurt, chia seeds, pumpkin, sesame, peanut, etc., spinach butter

c) Low carb vegan

Micronutrients; vitamins

Vegan LCHF diet prompts

a) Eliminate grain, eliminate/limit legumes (good iron and protein sources)

b) Eliminate/limit fruits

c) Add more low carb high protein e.g. tofu, nuts seed, low-carb high-fat seeds, nuts, avocado tahini. Add fat boosters, oils and iron booster, seeds and green leafy vegetables, add micronutrient boosters without added sugar.

Vegan LCHF non-haem iron sources: high vitamin C foods increase the absorption of non-haem iron.

Half capsicum=200% RDI Vitamin C.

LCHF and Irritable Bowel Syndrome (IBS):
Patients with Irritable bowelSyndrome (IBS)who are on a LCHF diet have specific challenges. At the start of the LCHF Program, some patient's gut

symptoms improve while other patient's gut problems are aggravated e.g bloating, diarrhea, pain, wind (offensive), constipation, gurgling, and cramping which are managed by avoiding foods high in FODMAPS.

Patients should be encouraged to consume nuts, almond milk, probiotics, and yogurts and avoid sugar. They should also increase berries e.g. strawberries, avocado, mushroom, and cream butter.

Not losing weight on LCHF: If there is no weight loss while on LCHF you should do calorie count.

*DR Andreas Eenfeldt: Maintaining weight loss and type-2 diabetes reversal: (173):*Low carb is real food and is sustainable for life which is almost opposite of Conventional Dietary Advice which from 1984 in the USA has led to obesity which has tripled rates in one generation.

Diabetes was at 10% of the population in 2010. There is no significant evidence for concluding that dietary saturated fat is associated with an increased risk of CVD or CHD.

Replacing saturated fats (SFA) with mostly polyunsaturated fats (PUFA) is unlikely to reduce CHD events, CHD mortality or total mortality. These findings have implications for the Current Dietary Recommendation. RCTS comparing low carb and low-fat diet on weight loss and CVD risk factors show that low carb diets have more weight loss, reduced blood pressure and CVD risk but slightly high LDL-c. Low carb diets lead to higher metabolic rates leading to more weight loss without counting calories and reversal of diabetes.

Sustainability of keto diets:
LCHF Ketogenic diets are sustainable for long durations according to different low carb diet studies e.g. 6 months Westman trials, 12 months: Hallberg, and 44 months: Nielson. "Patients have reversed diabetes for 15 years" (Dr Ted Neiman, and Dr Jay Wortman).

The side effects of LCHF diets initially are minor: keto flu, leg cramps, constipation, bad breath, heart palpitations, reduced physical performance, elevated cholesterol which is usually not an issue but improved HDL and triglycerides.

No supplements are needed in the Ketogenic diets; BUY REAL FOODS.
The study which showed that low carbohydrate intake is associated with high mortality is a prospective cohort study, and meta-analysis was not scientifically done and it is not valid.

"Nutritional epidemiology is a Scandal; it should just go to the dustbin" Prof John Loannides.

Red meat and Health: Nina Teicholz (174)

There has been biasing against red meat especially by Vegans e.g. Red meat and disease outcomes like diabetes, cancer, and heart disease. Red meat consumption has gone down but diabetes prevalence has gone up.

Meat and colorectal cancer: A 2015 study showed an association of processed meat, red meat and colorectal cancer.

1. The limitation of this study is that it is based on epidemiology, which is a very weak kind of science that can only show association, not causation.
2. An association in epidemiology can be considered as "cause and effect" if it meets certain criteria, the most important of which is the 'Strength of association'.
3. Compare that number 1.17 'relative risk' for fresh meat and cancer and 1.18 'relative risk' for processed meat and cancer.

An example of a strong association is smoking and lung cancer. Heavy smokers had a 15-30 times greater risk of dying of lung cancer v/s never smokers.

Relative risks of less than 2 are unreliable. People who eat red meat are likely to have other unhealthy behaviors e.g. high body fat, waist circumference, BMI, lower education, physical inactivity, and smokers, and more alcohol drinking. Epidemiology relies on self-reported data which is notoriously unreliable.

Clinical trials on red meat and cancer

1. **Polyp Prevention Trial:** the patient had a significant decrease in red and processed meats and results showed no recurrence of cancerous polyps. Relative risk of 1.0.

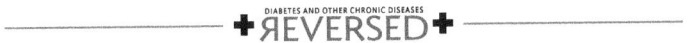
2. **Women Health Initiative**: 8-year follow-up on a diet with reduced red meat by 20%, showed no effect on colorectal cancer.

What were the proposed mechanisms for red meat causing cancer? Is it Heme iron 80% blood or N-nitroso-compounds which are said to be carcinogenic? But there should be guidelines on declaring what is carcinogenic.

Red meat and heart disease are not correlated: Red meat consumption has dropped and yet the prevalence of heart disease has not dropped. Saturated fats and cholesterol were the original reason that red meat was thought to cause heart disease and this has been proved not to be true. Where is the effect of saturated fats on cardiovascular mortality or total mortality?

Red meat and heart disease: a meta-analysis of randomized controlled trials that compare the lipid effects of beef v/s poultry and or fish consumption concluded that the changes in fasting lipid profile were not significantly different from beef consumption compared with those with poultry and fish consumption.

Total red meat intake of 20.5 serving per day dose does not relatively influence cardiovascular disease risk factors (i.e. lipids and lipoproteins), shows a systematically searched meta-analysis of Randomized Controlled Trials.

Research by Rashmi Sinha still believes red meat causes cancer. *Meat intake and Mortality: (175),* the Cohort Study was done by estimating meat intake from a food frequency questionnaire, concluded that red and processed meat intakes were associated with modest increases in total cancer and CVD mortality.

The mechanism of red meat causing cancer through nitrate/nitrite is controversial since human exposure to nitrate is mainly exogenous through the consumption of vegetables and to a lesser extent water and other foods. Nitrate is also formed endogenously. In contrast, exposure to its metabolite nitrite is mainly from endogenous nitrate conversion *(176).*

Weak science promoted by Activist groups and special interests (animal welfare groups) are pushing for the elimination of all types of animal food. This is coupled by the environmental group's propaganda that eating red meat encourages global warming.

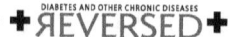

Some vegetarian diet doctors are active and well-funded by some carbohydrate companies.

Summary

"There is no evidence that red meat is bad for health. Weak science is being promoted, driven by ideological activists and bias among academicians. Consensus and repetition do not make weak evidence strong" Nina Teicholz.

Conclusion
Although the animals (livestock) increase the production of carbon dioxide and methane resulting in 0.36% of greenhouse gas emissions globally and are blamed for depletion of the ozone layer and climate change, keeping of livestock and applying good agricultural practices naturally restores soil fertility leading to better environmental conservation **(171)**.

There are also options for Vegans or Vegetarian LCHF diets which can have adequate nutrients with the proper advice from a qualified Nutritionist/Dietician. Patients with Irritable Bowel Syndrome (IBS) can also be advised on the right LCHF diet **(172)**.

KEY TAKEAWAYS:
- *Many social challenges should be considered in LCHF diet implementation.*
- *LCHF diet is a sustainable lifestyle.*
- *Good agricultural practices in keeping livestock naturally restores soil fertility and does not significantly contribute to climate change*
- *Vegan LCHF diet is available.*
- *No supplements are needed in LCHF diet.*
- *Ignore some prospective cohort studies.*
- *Red meat is not correlated to heart disease and cancer*

CHAPTER THIRTY

LCHF DIET AND PREGNANCY

Perhaps there is no issue in the LCHF diet as heated and controversial as the LCHF during pregnancy.

CASE 1

A 31-year-old woman who had Precocious Puberty at 3 years, and Polycystic Ovary Syndrome (PCOS) at 14, weight gain to 145 kg, height 183cm and prediabetes by 20 years and she was infertile, adopted a LCHF diet, lost 54 kg, established regular periods, blood glucose normalized, ovaries reduced and depression was uplifted. She became pregnant and continued with a LCHF diet during pregnancy and gave birth to healthy twins.

Ketones in urine scare many doctors into fearing life-threatening ketoacidosis in pregnancy or starvation ketosis. The small number of Primary Care Doctors and Obstetricians/Gynecologists who understand are comfortable with Nutritional Ketosis.

Few studies if any enroll pregnant mothers because of liability, ethical concerns and the physiological complexity of pregnancy. Evidence-Based Medicine (EBM) about what is best for pregnant mothers is lacking. It is well known from increasing long term Observation Studies that unique physiological condition and complications of pregnancy predict future risks in both mother and their offspring e.g. Gestational Diabetes.

Fostering a healthy pregnancy is paramount for mother and child. In this research vacuum many doctors default to the recommended advice; eat low fat with plenty of fruit and healthy grains. Some even become hysterical if a pregnant mother says she is on a LCHF diet. They say; "You are harming your baby" citing research in mice that a ketogenic exposure in utero led to a smaller brain in development associated organ dysfunction and neurobehavioral changes when they become adult mice.

Effects of a ketogenic diet during pregnancy on embryonic growth in mice:
Dafna Sussman et al(177): The Gestational ketogenic diet deliriously affects maternal fertility and increases susceptibility to fetal ketoacidosis during lactation. Prenatal and early postnatal exposure to a ketogenic diet also results in significant alterations to neonatal brain structure and results in retarded physiological growth. These alterations could be accompanied by functional and behavioral changes in later postnatal life.

The above study finding is contrary to other studies that show an increase in ketone utilization enzymes within the brain during the second half of gestation, which is speculated to facilitate lipid and myelin (white matter) synthesis favorable for the developing Brain.

Use of LCHF in gestational diabetes, preeclampsia, hyperemesis gravidarum, pregnancy in DMT2: "It is completely safe for women to be eating a ketogenic diet in pregnancy according to **Michael Fox, a Fertility Specialist at Jacksonville Centre for Reproductive Medicine** who has been recommending LCHF for 17 years to his infertile patients but also to all his patients who become pregnant". He has had hundreds of patients who have been completely ketotic throughout pregnancy without any untoward effects. He recommends the women to start a LCHF diet 2 or 3 months before trying to conceive so that the mother is adapted before entering pregnancy. Once pregnant, the mother enjoys frequent low carb high fat eating every two hours from the time she wakes up with no fasting. He provides a dietary handout with listed food items for meals and snacking e.g. cream, nuts, vegetables, eggs, etc.

In his experience eating this way decreases rates of miscarriage, preeclampsia, gestational diabetes and hyperemesis gravidarum. "Nausea is a reactive hypoglycemic reaction to the dramatically increased Insulin resistance caused by pregnancy hormones," he said. Ketogenic diet relieves this hypoglycemia associated with Insulin resistance".

DR Robert Kiltz a Fertility Specialist at "CNY Fertility" has been recommending the ketogenic diet for improved fertility for the last 5 years. He highly supports LCHF foods during conception and pregnancy. "We have zero

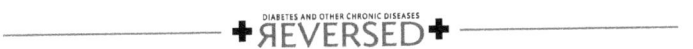

need for carbohydrates as humans". Despite witnessing many keto successful pregnancies he is still a minority of Fertility Doctors who recommend this approach.

Ketogenic expert, author Maria Emmerich has counseled hundreds of women on ketogenic eating during pregnancy with great results. "As if this diet of real food would be harmful to the fetus," She asks while pointing out that the fetus is naturally in a frequent state of ketosis, and that it is necessary for "laying down fatty structures like brain and nerve cells".

Another expert in low carb or ketogenic diets in pregnancy is *US Dietician Lily Nichols* whose popular books *"Real Food for Pregnancy (178) and Real Food for Gestational Diabetes (179)"* has a whole chapter on the misconceptions surrounding ketosis in pregnancy. She has helped hundreds of pregnant women in her career as a Specialist in Gestational Diabetes (GD) also known as "carbohydrate intolerance in pregnancy". GD is important in women with undiagnosed prediabetes prior to pregnancy. "I find it ironic that if you tell your doctor that you plan to eat low carb during pregnancy they will say it is unsafe, but if you say you plan to eat fresh vegetables, meat, fish, eggs, dairy, nuts, seeds and little fruit they will tell you to stay on course.''

Is the low carb high fat safe during pregnancy? Lily Nichols:(180) "We are trained on Government Guidelines. There is a misconception about saturated fat, animal fat and full-fat dairy products. *Real food is unprocessed foods, meats, fish, dairy, nuts, and seeds*. Pregnancy guidelines have an imbalance in macronutrient ratio. They are low in fat, protein and very high in carbs. The carbs should be low especially for patients with GD. Pregnant women are advised to avoid many foods during pregnancy due to safety issues since there is reduced susceptibility to infection due to lowered immunity during pregnancy e.g. Listeria/Salmonella but avoiding the foodstuffs may lead to a deficiency of some nutrients. You should be moderately conscious than avoiding the foods.

Eating of well-prepared raw fish (Sushi), cheese, eggs is permitted. Cravings during pregnancy are triggered by high carb diets e.g. breakfast.
Eating small frequent meals should be individualized. Intermittent fasting is not advisable.

Is low carb safe during pregnancy? Lily Nichols: Mothers with GD have a 19 times higher chance of the child developing diabetes. In the USA in 2014, the total carbohydrate recommended for pregnant women is more than 300gm per day. In most of the GD patients, glucose control gets worse. Standard carbohydrate recommendations for pregnant women are 45-60% carbs with a minimum of 175gm/day carbs. Conventional GD meal plan is 227gm carbs/day, 45-60gm carbs lunch and 30gm carbs dinner.

Total grand carb per day is 175gm but the lower limit of dietary carbs compatible with life apparently is zero, provided that adequate amounts of protein and fat are consumed. The marginal amount of carbs required in the diet in an energy balanced state is conditional and dependent upon the remaining composition of the diet.

Ketones are erroneously considered unsafe during pregnancy. In some instances women may be eating the right amount and type of carbohydrate foods for their bodies but still have high blood glucose levels. If this happens it is important to cut back on carbohydrates and not to give Insulin.

"Inadequate carbohydrate intake can result in ketosis which may harm fetal development": This is a disputed result of an old study in mice. Women in labor have ketones due to poor eating.

As part of adaptation to pregnancy, there is a decrease in maternal blood glucose concentration, development of Insulin resistance and a tendency to develop ketosis. Maternal ketone bodies level increase in gestation 2-3 fold from baseline and the relative Insulin resistance also gradually increases with gestational time resulting in susceptibility to a ketotic state. Therefore ketosis happens naturally in pregnancy.

Types of ketosis are rarely differentiated but they are important in understanding risks/benefits.

Nutritional ketosis, starvation ketosis, diabetic ketoacidosis

    a) In nutritional ketosis, the body burns primarily fat for fuel because the diet is limited in carbohydrates but not energy due to adequate calories from fat and protein. Blood sugar remains normal. Benign nutritional ketosis is the state that pregnant women often experience when eating a lower carb, calorie appropriate diet.

ii) In starvation ketosis, the body is burning primarily stored body fat for fuel because the person is eating inadequate calories from all sources. By definition maternal diet is depleted in essential fatty acids, amino acids, vitamins, minerals, micronutrients, and antioxidants. It is unsafe because calorie restriction profoundly alters the levels of amino acids in amniotic fluid.

iii) Diabetic ketoacidosis (DKA) occurs in Type-1 diabetes or in Insulin-dependent Type-2 diabetes due to inadequate exogenous Insulin (pregnancy is naturally hyperinsulinemic). Blood sugar levels are 3 times normal. There is an incorrect acid-base balance (acidic blood PH), very high blood ketones (10-20mmols/L). It is extremely unsafe and may harm fetal neuropsychomotor development.

Ketones in urine do not mean the patient is in DKA.

	Nutritional Ketosis (safe)	Starvation Ketosis (unsafe)	Diabetic Ketoacidosis (unsafe)
Blood glucose	normal	normal/low	high
Urine ketones	present	absent	present
Blood ketones	absent/trace	low	very high
Blood PH	normal	Acidic	extremely acidic
Nutritional intake	Adequate calories/[ow carb	Inadequate calories from all sources	N/A

NB. In pregnancy urine ketones DO NOT correlate with blood ketone levels, only blood ketones are clinically relevant. Low-level ketosis is normal. Compared to non-pregnant women, healthy pregnant women have blood ketones 3-fold higher in the morning.

Healthy pregnant women show a marked elevation of ketones after 12-18 hour fast. Four hours after a meal the ketones will be in the range of nutritional ketosis (0.3-4mmol/L).

In late pregnancy, catabolism makes ketosis even more frequent.

In early pregnancy, the body is in an anabolic state (lower Insulin resistance), programmed to build maternal fat stores, aside from nausea/food aversions, the mother is less prone to ketosis.

Late pregnancy is catabolic (higher insulin resistance), programmed to shunt nutrients to the baby, including mobilizing maternal fat stores and are more prone to ketosis.

Theories for higher ketone levels:
1.   Brain development: fetal brain gets 30% of its energy from ketones. Ketones are used to synthesize essential cerebral lipids.
2.   Energy in late pregnancy: maternal generation of ATP comes from almost exclusively from burning fats.
3.   Infant survival: healthy infants Exclusively Breastfed (EBF) stays in ketosis for at least the first month of life. *(Glycative Stress Response 2016).*

Another theory is that high blood sugar is risky leading to congenital heart defects, Neural Tube Defects (NTDs), spinal defects, and malformations of kidneys and (even below GD levels). Other congenital malformations associated with high blood sugar are cleft palate, limb reduction defects, polydactyly (extra fingers/toes), enlarged pancreas which leads to 6 times the risk of DMT2 by age 13, and Stillbirth. Maybe that is why blood sugar in healthy women is always 20% lower during pregnancy.

HAPO study involving 25000 women showed the risk of elevated blood sugar is continuous, resulting in more Macrosomia, Cesarean sections, and Post-delivery hypoglycemia in babies.

Fetal programming (Epigenetics):

1. Maternal hyperglycemia leads to Leptin dysregulation, impaired methylation; likely contributing to long term programming of excessive adiposity later in life, hyperinsulinemia and pancreatic hyperplasia.
2. High GI diet in pregnancy is associated with metabolic syndrome in offspring at age 20 years.

Problems with high carb:

1. Carbohydrates lead to higher blood sugar, higher insulin levels, and more fat storage.
2. Amniotic fluid Insulin levels, which reflect fetal pancreatic /Insulin production, correlate with obesity during adolescence.
3. Maternal carbohydrate intake (especially sugar) is an independent risk factor for childhood obesity.

Current health crisis:

1. 2/3 women of reproductive age are overweight or obese.
2. 18% of pregnant women have gestational diabetes (carbohydrate intolerance).
3. Excess weight and excess blood sugar are by far the most common causes of excess fetal growth (macrosomia).
4. Childhood obesity and diabetes are on the rise.

Should we be eating so many carbs?

Estimation of carb intake in 229 Hunter-Gatherer diets worldwide is approximately 16-22% calorie is carbs, closer to Equator people have higher carb (30-35%) and closer to Poles lower carbs (less than 15%). Most ancestral foods are less "carbohydrate-dense").

Carb quantity: The average prenatal diet is 2400-2600 calories, conventional recommendations are 45-65% carbs (270-420gm), compared with hunter-gatherer intake 16-22% (96-143gm) or extreme latitudes (Inuit of Alaska) 3-15% carbs (18-98gm).

Nutrient density v/s carbohydrate quality: A higher glycemic load diet is associated with poorer nutrient intake in women with GD, and higher dietary GI and GL are most predictions of inadequate micronutrient intake in pregnancy. Diets high in grains are linked to excess infant birth weight.

There is better sugar control in a low glycemic diet which has been shown to lower the chance of requiring Insulin in GD pregnancy by 50%.
A low glycemic index diet attenuates typical Insulin resistance seen in late pregnancy. Eating nuts, avoiding juice, cereals, and cookies leads to a reduced risk of GD.

Healthier children: Low GI diet in pregnancy has a beneficial effect on neonatal central adiposity and Low GI in the 3rd trimester and has less chance of excess adiposity of the infant at 6 months.

Optimal carbohydrate intake in pregnancy

1. 90-150gm per day total carb, meeting micronutrient needs, and blood glucose regulation should be given priority.
2. Emphasize low-glycemic nutrient-dense carbs like non-starchy vegetables, nuts, seeds, Greek yogurt, and berries, etc.
3. There is variable tolerance for starchy carbs, fruit, and adequate physical activity. Weight gain, blood sugar/pressure are avoided. Opt for low carb breakfast since Insulin resistance (IR) tends to be higher in the morning.
4. Personalize to the client: low carb is not no or zero carb. Even if you eat low carb you will likely still eat carbohydrates. Depending on the carb tolerance, higher carb foods can still be eaten in moderation, such as whole grains, legumes, and starchy vegetables. The goal is to eliminate refined grains and cut way back on sugar.

Key nutrient-dense foods are naturally low carb e.g. liver, organ meats, meat on bone, slow-cooked meat, bone broth, eggs, full fat, and fermented dairy products, fatty fish, sea vegetables, and green leafy vegetables.

Example	Standard Conventional American Diet	LCHF Diet: Eat Real Food
Breakfast	Oatmeal, strawberry Low-fat milk	Eggs, cooked butter, mushroom Tangerine
Lunch/Dinner	Chicken sandwich Banana, low-fat milk	Grass-fed beef, spaghetti Tomato, brocoli, cream cheese
Snack	Carrot slices, whole wheat cruncher	full-fat yogurt, berries
Dessert	Low-fat frozen yogurt	dark chocolate/cashew nuts

Conclusion
1. A nutrient-dense, real food prenatal diet reduces the risk for mother and baby.
2. Carb needs will vary from woman to woman but are generally lower than conventional guidelines.
3. Emphasize nutrient-dense, low-GI carbs, vegetables, whole fruit, nuts, and seeds.
4. Low-level ketosis is a natural part of pregnancy.

For some women who in the early days of pregnancy feel better eating slightly more carbs, go for it but opt for nutrient-dense foods. All women benefit from the most nutrient-dense diet they can manage and just happen to be naturally lower in carbohydrates.

Taking a LCHF diet during pregnancy is associated with normal blood pressure, moderate weight gain and normal babies delivered. "Don't say keto, say you are eliminating sugar and processed starchy foods. No doctor is going to give you a daily sugar requirement".

KEY TAKEAWAYS:
1. *Having ketones in urine during pregnancy is normal.*
2. *A LCHF diet is eating real food, in pregnancy.*

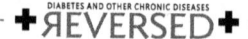

3   *A low Glycaemic Index diet in pregnancy can lower insulin requirement in gestational diabetes by 50%*

4   *A LCHF diet in pregnancy is associated with normal blood pressure, moderate weight gain and normal babies.*

All women benefit from the most nutrient-dense diet they can manage and just happen to be naturally lower in carbohydrates.

CHAPTER THIRTY ONE

LOW CARBOHYDRATE KETOGENIC DIET AND BREASTFEEDING (LACTATION)

Not a lot of scientific studies have been done on the effect of LCHF ketogenic diet on breastfeeding; however, studies from lactating women in the USA and Sweden *(181)* concluded that women can successfully breastfeed their infants if they have been provided calorie intakes of 1800-2200 Kcal/ day. Collectively these observations indicate that the intake recommended by the Institute of Medicine during the first six months-*Estimated energy requirement plus 400Kcal/day for lactating women (182)* may be in significant excess of their true needs and should women accurately follow these recommendations, it might hinder their ability to lose weight in the postpartum period. Obesity is an increasingly serious health concern. There is evidence that excessive postpartum weight retention contributes to the development of obesity *(183), (184)* and obesity-related diseases. The use of low calorie and low carbohydrate diet to facilitate weight loss during lactation could result in reduced milk production, elevated plasma lipid, prolonged ketosis and diet-related deficiencies in micronutrient and fiber.

However, published studies have compared the effects of low carbohydrate diets on maternal health and or milk volume and composition.

Numerous metabolic adaptations occur during lactation to support milk synthesis without jeopardizing maternal substrate homeostasis while optimizing the delivery of appropriate amounts of substrates for the sucking infant.

Lactating women have a glucose production rate greater than 35% higher than that of the control of non-lactating women. This elevated glucose production results from high rate gluconeogenesis and hexoneogenesis (lactose derived from glucose and galactose) within the breast.

In the 2009 Study: *Effect of dietary macronutrient composition under moderate hypocaloric intake on maternal adaptation during lactation: Mahmoud A*

Mohammad et al (185) A group of lactating mothers were compared, on one occasion receiving high fat (30%), carb (55%) and on the second occasion receiving high carb (60%), (25%) fat. Milk production, infant intakes, and substrate and hormone concentrations were measured. Glucose rates of appearance, production, gluconeogenesis, glycogenolysis, and hexoneogenesis were measured.

The study showed that the macronutrient composition under isonitrogenous, isocaloric conditions of maternal diet had no short-term effect on milk volume or its aqueous components protein and lactose.

High-fat diet increased milk fat concentration and content by 13% and 15% respectively, when compared with the high carb diet. This increased the calorie content of the milk. This increase in milk fat led to increased fat and calorie intake by the infant. These findings agree with those of *Park et al (186)*, who reported that women who consumed a diet low in dairy fat had lower milk fat than when they consumed more dairy fat.

In moderate caloric restriction, overall milk production and milk energy output were comparable with published values for well-nourished women *(187)*

Dusdieker L B: Is milk production impaired by dieting during lactation? (188). "This study was to determine the weight loss program during lactation. The findings suggest that modest weight loss by healthy breastfeeding women does not adversely affect either quantity or quality of milk consumed by their infants.

Both glucose concentrations and glucose production rates were higher with the high carb diet than with high fat. The insulin and C-peptide in the high carb diet were higher than those with the high-fat diet.

Lactating mothers who consumed a high-fat diet decreased carbohydrate oxidation but increased fat oxidation leading to higher plasma free fatty acids and *beta*-hydroxybutyrate concentrations.

In conclusion, under moderate calorie restriction, milk production was not affected by maternal diet composition. *Milk fat, energy content and infant energy intake were higher during the higher fat diet.* The lactating mothers adapted

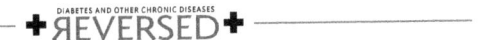
increased glucose demand and low carbohydrate intake via decreased glucose oxidation but not via increased glucose production.

Additional studies are warranted to determine whether a hypocaloric higher fat diet might promote greater weight loss during lactation than would a high carb diet while maintaining sufficient milk production.

The 2016 literature review by ***Braier F et al "Impact of maternal nutrition on breast milk composition: A systematic review": (189)*** It is reported that maternal diet influences the nutritional composition of breast milk. The amount of variability in human milk attributable to diet remains mostly unknown. Most original studies that reported a dietary influence on breast milk composition did not assess diet directly, did not qualify its association with milk composition or both, 36 publications were identified.

Brewer M M: PostPartum changes in maternal weight and body fat deposits v/s non-lactating mothers: (190) Maternal weight and body fat changes in 56 women were studied from delivery to 6 months postpartum breastfeeding (lactating) or/and formula feeding combination. Results suggest lactation plays a role in Post-partum weight and body fat loss but the current RDA may be too high to permit such loses.

Lovelady C A et al: The effect of weight loss in overweight lactating women on the growth of their infants: (191) the retention of weight during pregnancy may contribute to obesity and lactation may promote weight loss. This study concluded that weight loss of approximately 0.5 kg per week between 4 and 14 weeks post-partum in overweight women who exclusively breastfeed does not affect the growth of their infants.

Conclusions:
"The available information on this topic is scarce and diversified. Most of the evidence currently used in clinical practice to make recommendations is limited to studies that only reported indirect associations".

Therefore, maternal nutrition has little or no effect on many nutrients in human milk, for others, human milk may not be designed as a primary nutritional source

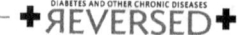
for the infant and for a few, maternal nutrition can lead to substantial variations in human milk quality.

Study on the impact of maternal diet in human milk composition and neurological development of infants: Innis S M (192) got inconsistent findings. Human milk fatty acids are among the nutrients that show extreme sensitivity to maternal nutrition and are implicated in neurological development.

Maternal diet during pregnancy is relevant for fatty acids supply during fetal life and lactation for normal growth of Brain and visual system.

The study on **"maternal diet during pregnancy and lactation on the fatty acid composition of erythrocytes and breast milk of Chilean women': Barera et al(193)** concludes that it is necessary to increase the intake of polyunsaturated fatty acids (PUFA) especially omega 3 & 6 fatty acids during pregnancy and lactation by improving the quality of consumed foods with particular emphasis on omega 3 content.

"Maternal diet and nutrient requirements in pregnancy and breastfeeding: An Italian Consensus Document by Marangoni Franca 2016: (194) shows that very hard scientific evidence supports the importance of lifestyle and dietary habits (with adequate micronutrient intake) during pregnancy and breastfeeding for the health status of the women and their offspring.

The consumption of a varied and balanced diet from preconception period is essential to ensure maternal wellbeing and favorable outcome of pregnancy. Even in most Industrialized Countries specific dietary intakes in pregnancy and lactation are often inadequate. With respect to the Italian population, the available data indicates that the intake of selected nutrients in selected population groups (Vegan and/or Vegetarian exclusion of eggs, milk, and meat) and in pregnant and lactating women can be inadequate. This particularly applies to DHA (omega 3), iodine, iron, calcium, folic acid, and vitamin D.

Therefore, with the currently available information, it is not possible to talk about the effects of LCHF ketogenic diet on lactation (breastfeeding) with certainty.

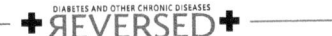

Some tips for breastfeeding while following a ketogenic diet by *DR Antony Gustin: August 2018:*

1. Start the ketogenic diet early. For some patients with PCOS, this will increase the chance of pregnancy.
2. Avoid dehydration.
3. Don't forget your nutrients and electrolytes.
4. Consume enough calories especially high-quality fats.
5. Consume enough fiber and vegetables.
6. Try a moderately low carb diet. Rather than strict keto (50-75gm carbs/day).
7. Track your food/drink consumption and daily milk production.

"If you are breastfeeding, you should not do a strict low carb diet. You need to add more carbs to be safe (choose a moderately low carb diet with at least 50gm carbs/day. It will still be effective" DR Andreas Eenfeldt M.D. 2019.

KEY TAKEAWAYS:

- *A low calorie, low carbohydrate diet may facilitate weight loss during lactation*
- *LCHF diet increases breast milk fat leading to increased fat and calorie intakes for the infant.*

"*Maternal diet during pregnancy is relevant for fatty acids supply during fetal life and lactation for normal growth of Brain and visual system.*"

CHAPTER THIRTY TWO

ROLE OF SWEETENERS IN DIABETES MANAGEMENT

A sweetener is a sugar substitute (a food additive that provides a sweet taste like that of sugar while containing significantly less food energy than sugar-based sweetener, making it a zero-calorie or low calorie-sweeteners).

Although in the principles of dietary management of DMT2, *(35), (172)"It states clearly that sweeteners are not* **essential** *and should be avoided as much as possible, there is widespread use of sweeteners by diabetics"*. Sweeteners are used to stop sugar cravings or as part of dietary advice by Healthcare Educators. Statements like "diet coke and artificial sweetener tablets are safe for diabetics instead of sugary beverages or sugarless tea" are common. Incidents of DMT2 continue to rise and reduction in obesity; one of the main factors linked to DMT2 is a priority in the prevention and management of DMT2.

Low-calorie sweeteners (LCS) may provide an alternative to sugar and may facilitate weight loss or maintenance by limiting caloric intake. In the ***role of LCS in diabetes: Craig A Johnson et al (195)*** describes reasons for use of LCS:

1. Reduction in caloric intake as an alternative way of managing obesity.
2. Treatment of diabetes since they are assumed not to raise blood glucose and are a practical way of reduction of carbohydrate intake.
3. Other benefits: Help in the reduction of dental caries.

The low-calorie sweetener has associated concerns: increased appetite, weight gain, increased Insulin, other hormonal responses and concerns e.g. allergic reactions.

Conclusion:
Although the use of LCS in the treatment of diabetes and obesity may be promising, high quality clinical human research is needed.

DR Doron Sher an Orthopedic Surgeon: Artificial Sweeteners (196) gives a very informative lecture on sweeteners covering; Classification, details of common sweeteners, the risk associated with sweeteners, risk of DMT2, CHD, and cancer.He starts by saying that bitter things are generally poisonous while sweet things are nutritionally dense and we tend to eat them. Taste is the sensation that is produced when a substance chemically interacts with taste cells in the mouth (tongue) which sends signals to the brain. Saliva dissolves the food because the smell is connected to taste. There are sweet receptors in other parts e.g. pancreas not only in the tongue. Bliss point depends on texture, feeling full and changes with the LCHF diet. The more Insulin, the more the desire for sweet foods; glucagon enhances taste reception.

The brain responds with a reward and there is habitual stimulation of reward pathway mediated through dopamine and these are the same pathways to addictive substances and relative sweetness. Obese people need more stimulation and more sugar to get the same response.

Categories of sweeteners
1. Origin: natural or artificial
2. Technical qualities: sweetness, after taste, solubility, stability, and ability to be cooked.
3. Nutritional value: caloric v/s non-caloric, digestibility, and sweetness potency.

Sweeteners can be classified into:
1. Sugars
2. Sugar alcohols (nutritive)
3. Natural caloric sweeteners
4. Artificial sweetener (non-nutritive).

No added sugar mostly means high fructose.
1. Sugars: maltose, sucrose, fructose, etc.
2. Sugar alcohols; sorbitol, erythritol, and xylitol are mainly found naturally in fruits and vegetables but are mainly and easily processed from other sugars and they are not digestible. They are used in chocolate, jelly, and sweets.

The Insulin response to maltitol, sorbitol and xylitol is half the response of sugar and they increase insulin metabolic response (Insulin Resistance).

Erythritol gives mild insulin response, causes dose-dependent GI responses and appears safe unless you are metabolically unwell.

3. Natural caloric sweeteners: Stevia is derived from a South American shrub and is found as an extract or a white powder that is derived from leaves. It is purchased commercially in extract, powder or in a powdered green herbal leaf.

It causes sweetness in a different pathway from sugar that is why it leaves a bitter after taste.

Beware: Stevia is often mixed with all sorts of sugars and sweeteners in the form of salts. Stevia causes no increase in blood glucose on its own and appears to increase insulin sensitivity in the pancreas. This may predispose to diabetic ketoacidosis.

Stevia is often combined with dextrose or maltodextrin to add bulk for cooking and these will raise insulin and blood sugar levels. Stevia has no positive side effects; it is approved for use as a sweetener by the joint Food and Agriculture Organization/WHO Expert Committee on Food and Additives 2005 and Generally Recognized as Safe (GRAS) approval from the Food and Drug Administration (FDA).

There are few studies on the effect on food intake and satiety levels, some studies point to effect on the gut microbiome, liver, and pancreatic stress.

Oligofructans (Chicory root) are bananas, onions, garlic, and blue agave. They resist intestinal breakdown, are fermented in the colon, and can diminish any aftertaste that can occur with other sweeteners. They cause no rise in blood sugar or insulin and are often combined with erythritol or Stevia.

1. Artificial sweeteners are high-intensity sweeteners, low-calorie sweeteners, and Artificially Sweetened Beverages (ASB). They are non-nutritive and provide a sweet sensation without altering blood sugar levels.

a) Organic acid derivatives: Saccharin, cyclamate, and Ace-k are polar synthetic compounds, not substrates for normal intermediate metabolism and not used as an energy source.

b) Peptides and peptide derivatives: Thaumatin and Aspartame. These are naturally occurring or metabolized food constituents, incorporated into intermediary metabolism used as energy sources, low-calorie applications arise from their intense sweetness.

Saccharin was the first artificial sweetener (1879) and it has been used since 1900-1970; it is FDA approved, it's not absorbed from or metabolized, it's 300 times sweeter than sugar, unstable when heated, no calories, does not increase glucose or blood sugar but it might stimulate an insulin response.

It is probably problematic in weight loss; it caused anemia, depressed growth, iron, vitamin A and folate deficiency, elevated Vitamin E in rats. It would seem reasonable to suggest that pregnant and breastfeeding mothers avoid them.

Cyclamate: sweetener code 952, it is 30-50 times sweeter than sucrose and often used with other artificial sweeteners. It is less expensive than most sweeteners, stable in heat, suitable for cooking and baking, was banned in the USA for safety concerns.

Acesulfame Potassium (Ace-k) is 200 times sucrose sweetness, aspartame, saccharin, and sucralose has a slightly bitter aftertaste, used in beverages has no carbohydrate. It has a stable BSL (no carbohydrate).

In rat studies: It significantly increases Insulin response and works directly on the pancreas and is not fully absorbed by the gut. Concerns have been raised about interaction with DNA potentially causing genetic damage in high doses. It is added to beverages e.g. coke zero.

Aspartame is the most popular artificial sweetener in use today. It is calorie and carbohydrate-free, great as a liquid sweetener. It is not ideal for cooking as it breaks down under high temperatures.

Aspartame was approved by the FDA and is used in over 6000 products. It is 200 times sweeter than sucrose and does not enter the bloodstream. It contains phenylalanine; care should be taken in phenylketonuria. Aspartame is hydrolyzed in the intestinal lumen into its components. It does not raise blood sugar and Insulin levels in humans.

Safety: Recent evidence demonstrates the effect on gut bacteria, changes in mitochondria with prolonged exposure, and stress responses affecting gluconeogenesis in the liver.

Phenylketonuria: beware and use in the short-term only.

Neotame is an Aspartame derivative; 30-60 times sweeter than Aspartame and 700-1300 times sweeter than sugar. It is eliminated via urine, non-caloric, caution in phenylketonuria

Sucralose is derived from regular sugar, not absorbed or recognized by the body. It has no calories. To crystalize it has to be bound to dextrose or maltodextrin and contains 0.5gram of carbohydrate per teaspoonful, it is 600 times sweeter than sugar. It causes Insulin response, weight gain or difficulty with weight loss when used in excess.

Trehalose is sugar; extracting it was difficult and costly. It lowers the freezing point of foods; used in ice creams.

Trehalose and C difficile: some strains of clostridium difficile in human gut microbiome are very responsive to Trehalose. It was introduced into the food supply in 2000. Hospitals acquired C difficile infections increased at about the same time.

Are artificial sweeteners safe?
1. Studies leading FDA approval have ruled out cancer risk.
2. Multiple study of Atherosclerosis:
3. Daily consumption of diet drinks is associated with a 36% greater risk of metabolic syndrome and a 67% increase in Type-2 diabetes.
4. Causes blood cancer: in rats in high doses.

How do they work: The relationship between research outcomes and risk of bias, study sponsorship, and author financial conflicts of interest in reviews of the effect of artificially sweetened beverages on weight outcomes: A systematic review of reviews showed BIAS.

Recent reviews of studies spanning at least the past 40 years have concluded that high-intensity sweeteners are potentially helpful, harmful, or have an as yet unclear effects with regard to regulation of energy balance and other metabolic consequences.

You say you can give up diet drinks whenever you want? Don't be sure.

Rats who are exposed to cocaine were given the choice between intravenous cocaine and oral saccharine; they chose saccharine, it gave them more dopamine response.

The San Antonio Heart Study: The risk of weight gain and obesity were significantly greater in those consuming artificially sweetened beverages (ASB) compared with those who did not consume ASB.

Increased risk of Type-2 diabetes with ASB/SSB:
1. Nurse's Health Study: Showed increased risk of DMT2 on consuming at least one ASB or Sugar-Sweetened Beverage (SSB) per day
   European Prospective Investigation into Cancer and Nutrition: Increased risk for DMT2 consuming one ASB or SSB per day even with normal weight at baseline.
2. Hypertension and cardiovascular disease: Risk of Coronary Heart Disease (CHD) was significantly elevated in multiple studies in people who consumed more than two ASB or SSB per day.
3. Diabetes: One serving of SSB per day leads to an 18% increase in DMT2. Adjusted to adiposity, association attenuated to 13%.

One serving ASB per day leads to a 25% greater incidence of DMT2, adjusted for adiposity, association attenuated to 8%.

One serving of fruit juice per day leads to a 7% incidence of DMT2

No benefit to using ASB or fruit juice over SSB.

There is a link between sweetness and calories. You crave more sweets, choose sweet foods over nutritious food and gain weight. Brain activation patterns in ASB drinkers showed that:

In people who drink ASB is different from brain activation to sucrose v/s humans who do not, and is the same brain activation pattern for saccharine and sucrose.

In people who don't drink ASB: different brain activation patterns for saccharine and sucrose.

There is an individual effect of sweeteners; between a metabolic syndrome person and a healthy athlete.

Avoiding sweeteners can lead to weight loss in obese patients.

Conclusion

There are really no healthy, inexpensive and safe sweeteners available that taste just like sugar.

Hormones and weight loss: weight is controlled by many hormones; Insulin may be the most important, Glucose stimulates insulin to rise, Keep the carbs low. Eat healthy whole foods, not sweeteners.

Anti-aspartame activists claim there is a link between Aspartame and a multitude of ailments including cancer, seizures, headache, depression, Attention Deficit Hyperactivity Disorder (ADHD), dizziness, weight gain, and birth defects.

Although all sweeteners should be discouraged, some sweeteners are generally recommended for a low carb diet; they have little or no sugar or calories i.e. Stevia, erythritol, sucralose, xylitol, monk fruit sweetener, and yacon syrup.

The following sweeteners are not ideal for a LCHF diet: Maltodextrin, honey, coconut sugar, maple syrup, agave nectar, and dates; they are high in sugar and carbohydrates.

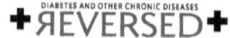
KEY TAKEAWAYS:

- *No sweetener is healthy, inexpensive and safe.*
- *Sweeteners are not essential*
- *Sweetened beverages are associated with DMT2, hypertension and obesity.*
- *Because of research bias, sweeteners can be helpful, harmful or have unclear effects.*

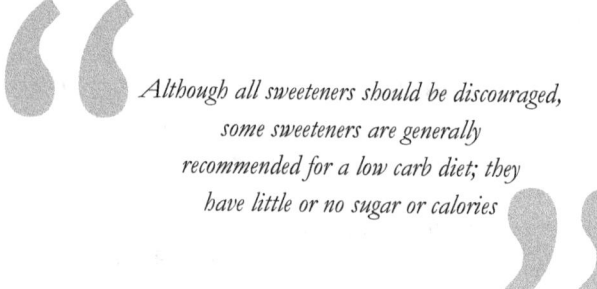

Although all sweeteners should be discouraged, some sweeteners are generally recommended for a low carb diet; they have little or no sugar or calories

CHAPTER THIRTY THREE

ANAESTHESIA AND LCHF DIET (KETOGENIC DIET)

L CHF ketogenic diet started being used in medical practice for nearly a century ago, mainly in the treatment of childhood epilepsy. The world is now embracing the use of these diets in the treatment of many Non-Communicable Diseases. Patients on these diets require anesthetic services and the Anesthetist/Anesthesiologist has to be aware of the unique challenges that are associated with the management of these patients i.e. Preoperative, Intraoperative and Postoperative Anesthetic Care.

A study done in the USA to determine if children on the ketogenic diet for management of epilepsy can safely undergo General Anesthesia (GA) for Surgical Procedures: *General anesthesia and the ketogenic diet: Clinical Experience in nine patients: Ignatio Valencia et al (197),* to determine if children on the ketogenic diet can undergo General Anesthesia (GA) for surgical procedures. The charts of children who had received GA while on the diet were evaluated with regard to demographics, procedure information, anesthesia records, blood chemistries, and perioperative course.

Of the 71 children on the KD during the period of study, nine (12.7%) had procedures requiring GA while on the diet. Nine children received GA for surgical procedures ranging from Central Line Placement to Hemispherectomy while on the KD. At the time of GA, the children ranged from 1 to 6 years and had been on the KD for 2 to 60 months. The patients received carbohydrate-free intravenous solutions peri-operatively.

Anesthesia duration ranged from 20 minutes to 11.5 hours. For longer procedures serum PH, glucose and electrolyte levels were monitored. Serum glucose levels remained stable in all patients but serum PH typically decreased, the largest reduction was to 7.16. In the three procedures patients received intravenous bicarbonate because of the level of acidosis. There were no perioperative complications.

Children on the KD can safely undergo GA for surgical procedures. Although serum glucose levels appear to be stable, serum PH or bicarbonate levels should be monitored because of the risk of metabolic acidosis.

Preoperatively, the diet was continued and blood chemistry i.e. glucose, *beta-hydroxybutyrate*, etc. were done. Intra-operatively, carbohydrate-free fluids e.g. normal saline or ringer's lactate were used. Blood glucose and blood gas analysis (BGA) and pH were monitored, and intraoperative bicarbonate was given intravenously to correct the metabolic acidosis noted in some procedures.

The inhalation induction of a pediatric epileptic patients on ketogenic diet with a high dose of Sevoflurane should be reconsidered due to epileptogenic potential of Sevoflurane:*Anesthetic management of a pediatric patient on a ketogenic diet: Ichikawa et al (198)* there are several specific considerations regarding seizure control during the perioperative period in patients who have been on a ketogenic diet (KD). A KD is high in fat, moderate in protein and low in carbohydrates and has a long history for the treatment of intractable seizures in children. Maintaining therapeutic ketosis and modifying the acid-base balance is particularly important for preventing seizures in patients on KD. This report shows changes in a patient with Double Cortex Syndrome who was on KD and who had been scheduled for the treatment of dental caries under sevoflurane anesthesia and acetate Ringer's administration.

*Diet-induced ketosis in epilepsy and anesthesia: Metabolic changes in three patients on a ketogenic diet: Hinton w et al (199)*ketogenic diets have high fat; moderate protein and low carbohydrate to induce ketosis which is monitored by daily urine testing. Lapses in diet control are frequently associated with loss of anticonvulsant control. There had never been a report of children maintained on a ketogenic diet subject to Anesthesia and Surgery.

This paper records the changes in metabolic variables observed in three patients undergoing simple inhalational anesthetics for minor surgery. All patients maintained low normal blood sugar concentrations and ketonemia during the preoperative period and induction of Anesthesia.

Glucose infusions were not given as this could have resulted in fall in plasma ketones and loss of seizure control.

There is a caution on the use of Enflurane in high concentrations and ketamine. *Fatal propofol infusion syndrome in association with ketogenic diet: Baumeister F A et al (200)* Propofol is used in refractory status epilepticus. When given as a long term infusion, propofol may cause a rare but frequently fatal complication; Propofol Infusion Syndrome (PIS).The hallmarks are metabolic acidosis, lipemia, rhabdomyolysis, and myocardial failure. PIS is caused by impaired fatty acid oxidation.

Ketogenic diet; high fat, moderate protein, and low carbohydrate diet is an effective treatment for difficult to control seizures. This is a report of a 10-year-old boy with catastrophic epilepsy who developed fatal infusion syndrome when a KD was initiated. Substances like propofol which impair fatty acid oxidation may pose a risk if combined with the ketogenic diet.

The induction and maintenance of GA with Propofol for a pediatric patient on a ketogenic diet is safe: *General Anesthesia with propofol for a paediatric patient on a ketogenic diet: Saito et al (201)*there are specific considerations regarding seizure control during the perioperative period in patients who are on a ketogenic diet (KD). The KD is a high fat, moderate protein, and low carb; it has a history of use for the treatment of intractable seizures in children. Maintaining ketosis and modifying the acid-base balance is particularly important for preventing seizures in patients on KD.

This is a report of a 3-year-old boy with seizures who was on KD and was scheduled for treatment of left Undescended Testis under Propofol Anesthesia and Ringers lactate. The induction and maintenance of anesthesia using Propofol was safe and reasonable for a patient on a KD.

In the short starvation preoperative period, sugary juices should not be given to the children on the ketogenic diet.

The Anesthetist/Anesthesiologist is likely to come across adults who are on LCHF ketogenic diets due to various diseases e.g. DMT1, DMT2, hypertension, epilepsy, polycystic ovary syndrome, chronic pain syndromes, chronic neurodegenerative disorders, old stroke, etc.

The Standard Anesthetic Protocol should be followed but remember the reduction in dietary carbohydrate intake leads to nutritional ketosis due to the

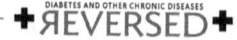
production of ketones which are used as an energy source instead of glucose. This relative but mild, safe acidotic state should be maintained preoperatively, intra-operatively and postoperatively. Intravenous fluids containing glucose e.g. 5% dextrose is discouraged.

Intraoperative blood glucose, BGA, pH, and ketones monitoring are encouraged in long operations. Normal saline is considered more beneficial than Ringer's lactate solution but normal saline should also be administered carefully because of the risk of exacerbating the patient's metabolic acidosis. One should be aware of the potential change of the ketogenic status due to drugs given intra-operatively.

Perioperative management of a pediatric patient on the ketogenic diet: James k Meneely (202) the ketogenic diet has become commonplace for the treatment of pediatric patients with refractory epilepsy. This article describes the perioperative management of a patient on KD. The basis, complications, and anesthetic implications of the diet are discussed. Postoperatively, patients should be back/continue with a LCHF diet as soon as possible.

Pediatric patients on ketogenic diet undergoing General Anesthesia (GA): A medical record Review: Soysal et al (203) the objective was to identify guidelines for anesthetic management and determine whether GA is safe for pediatric patients on KD. The study showed that it is relatively safe for children on KD to undergo GA. The three complications attributable to GA were mild and the increased seizure in two patients returned to baseline in 24 hours. Although normal saline is considered more beneficial than lactated Ringers solution in patients on KD, it should also be administered carefully because of the risk of exacerbating the patient's metabolic acidosis. One should be aware of the potential chance of the ketogenic status due to drugs given intra-operatively.

LCHF ketogenic diets can be used to prepare the grossly obese patients i.e. make the patient lose weight preoperatively and therefore make the patient suitable for bariatric surgery and anesthesia.

Very low carbohydrate before bariatric surgery: prospective evaluation of a sequential diet: Leonetti F et al (204) this was to evaluate the effectiveness of a sequential diet regimen termed Obese Preoperative Diet (OPOD) and a very low

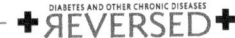
carbohydrate diet (VLCD) in morbidly obese patients with and without type-2 Diabetes Mellitus (DMT2) scheduled for Laparoscopic Bariatric Surgery. Bodyweight, body mass index, waist circumference, and neck circumference were significantly lower. In patients with DMT2 fasting blood glucose levels decreased significantly enabling the reduction of diabetic medications. Plasma and urine ketone levels increased but were less than 1mmol/litre and hunger decreased during the hunger period.

OPOD including a VLCKD was safe and effective in morbidly obese patients and it seems to be promising in these patients with and without DMT2 scheduled for laparoscopic bariatric surgery.

KEY TAKEAWAYS:

- *The preanaesthetic nutrition history of the patient is becoming more relevant*
- *Nutritional ketosis should be maintained during anaesthesia for patients on a LCHF diet.*
- *There are specific anesthetic considerations for patients on a LCHF diet.*

"
*In the short starvation preoperative period,
sugary juices should not be given to the children
on the ketogenic diet.*
"

CHAPTER THIRTY FOUR

MEDICOLEGAL ASPECTS OF PRESCRIBING LCHF KETOGENIC DIETS

The legal framework/laws vary from Country to Country but the principles are broadly similar.

1. International laws

2. National Constitution
   a. Criminal laws e.g. murder, manslaughter, grievous bodily harm, and health fraud.
   b. Civil law e.g. medical negligence, defamation, and libel.
   c. Administrative law e.g. licensing, health insurance, medical records, and data protection breaches, etc.
   d. Professional regulation e.g. registration, Code of Conduct, Clinical Guidelines, fitness to practice, professional hearings
   e. Registration and licensing

In Kenya, registration and licensing of doctors, hospitals and Medical Centers fall under the Medical Practitioners and Dentists Board. All other cadres of medical personnel involved in the implementation of the LCHF diet i.e Dieticians/Nutritionists, Nurses, Pharmacy and Laboratory Personnel must be licensed by their relevant Professional Bodies.

Professional Associations also issue professional rules/Ethics (by-laws) which must be complied with. Formulation and implementation of dietary interventions fall under the Kenya Nutritionists/Dieticians Act and a license from them is mandatory.

Other National and County laws must be followed and relevant Licenses obtained.

CIVIL LIABILITY

Medical Practitioners can be sued in court for damages due to medical negligence. Medical negligence refers to a breach of duty of care owed to a patient where an injury is directly caused by the breach.

The prescription of LCHF diets is increasing and extensive clinical trials have been done. The effectiveness of LCHF diets in refractory epilepsy and reversal of diabetes Type-2 is no longer debatable. There is a large International community and expanding list of countries including LCHF diets as a standard Medical option. Many systematic reviews have been done and International associations like the American Diabetic Association's recognition of the use of LCHF diets in the treatment of Diabetes Type-2 further confirms that prescribing a LCHF diet is within the Evidence-Based Medicine practiced worldwide.

Professional/medical negligence involves
  a) Duty of care: a patient must be in the care of a responsible Medical Practitioner
  b) Breach: this involves a breach of professional duty or Standard of Comparable Professional Practice.
  c) Did the Doctor act in accordance with a practice considered acceptable by a responsible Body of Doctors? And was the patient put into unnecessary risk? (Bolam or Bolitho Principle).

CRIMINAL/ADMINISTRATIVE LIABILITY

Medical Practitioners who engage in criminal activity can be prosecuted and sentenced in Court and administrative offenses e.g. offenses against privacy can arise.

The prescription of a LCHF diet can lead to the development of complications and may be viewed as a non-compliance with clinical guidelines in countries where LCHF diets have not been incorporated into the Standard Clinical Practice Guidelines (CPG). CPGs are defined as systematically developed statements to assist practitioner and patient decisions about appropriate health care for specific clinical circumstances. A deviation from the Evidence-Based Medicine (EBM) might make the clinician to be held accountable for poor outcome. EBM depends on clinical practice guidelines (CPGs) that have been developed, disseminated, and practiced.

How do evidence-based guidelines influence the determination of medical negligence? Hurwitz *(2004) (205)* "Guidelines do not actually set legal standards for clinical care but they provide the Courts with a benchmark by which to judge Clinical Conduct"

This article covers what is evidence-based guidance that worries clinicians, what is Medical Negligence, Guidelines, and the Courts, etc.

*Beyond the standard of care: A review model to judge medical negligence: Brenner L H et al: 2012 (206)*the standard of care has been used in law and medicine to determine whether medical care is negligent. However, the precise meaning of this concept is often unclear for both medical and legal professionals. *Conclusions: The standard of care is an inaccurate measure of medical negligence because it is premised on the faulty notion of conformity to norms.*

There are several clinical trials that show that prescribing LCHF diets is a more effective, less risky and cheaper approach than bariatric surgery in diabetes type-2 remissions.

An analysis of evidence-based medicine in the context of medical negligence litigation: Piennar 2011(207) "The use of forensic match evidence contains unavoidable paradox; that while it might be more reliable and precise than other forms of evidence, there exists a very real danger that Jurors will misapprehend its value given its quantitative nature".

Although there has not been a Court Case of a patient suing a Doctor for prescribing LCHF diets, it is necessary to be aware of the potential legal risks.

There are three high profile professional hearings against doctors since 2000:

1. *Annika Dahlqvist 2007 (prescribing LCHF diets to diabetes type-2/obese patient) (208)*
   Annika Dahlqvist the first Swedish LCHF pioneer ate low-fat, high-carb food according to the Dietary Guidelines. She became fatter and sicker and had fibromyalgia and Irritable Bowel Syndrome (IBS). She introduced herself to low-carb high-fat diet (LCHF) (saturated fat like butter and oils). She lost weight, got rid of fibromyalgia and IBS and was

very inspired and started the LCHF lifestyle message "if you are obese and or have type-2 diabetes you should eat LCHF diet: REAL NATURAL FOOD".

In 2005, two dietitians reported her to the Swedish National Board of Health and Welfare (NBHW) which deliberated for two years reviewing the science. They had the power to censure DR Dahlqvist or even revoke her medical license. In January 2008, they released their verdict: DR Dahlqvist had done nothing wrong. They stated: "low carbohydrate diet can today be seen as compatible with scientific evidence and best practice for weight reduction, Type-2 diabetes as several studies have shown in the short term and no evidence or harm has emerged!"

She continues to promote the LCHF lifestyle and that statins do more harm than good.

This was a revolutionary moment in Sweden and the verdict resulted in huge headlines. The low carbohydrate diet instantly went from being considered a dangerous "fad diet" to something that was proven to work and to some extent, officially endorsed by Government.

DR Eenfeldt popularized the diet in Scandinavia with his book *"The Food Revolution"*. In 2016 LCHF was the most popular diet as Sweden's statistics on obesity, heart disease, and cardiovascular risks have been going down.

2. AHPRA VS Gary Fettke 2014 (Lack of qualification to advise patients on nutrition) (209)
DR Gary Fettke an orthopedic surgeon was tired of amputating patient's limbs. He had been recommending low-carb diets to obese and Type-2 diabetes patients for two years. The Australian Health Practitioner Regulation Agency (AHPRA) decided to silence him.

DR Fettke had researched a lot about LCHF diets and his patients greatly benefited from his advice and the diet reportedly caused no harm to any of them.

AHPRA considered that Fettke was not an expert in the field of nutrition and had no authority to give such advice.

Chief among complaints was that he advised LCHF diets to patients with obesity and Type-2 Diabetes (DMT2). The dieticians claimed that LCHF was "inappropriate" advice and not evidence-based. They also claimed it was "inconsistent" with Australia's Heart Foundation position statement on dietary fats.

A Senate Enquiry in 2016 brought AHPRA's action under special scrutiny. DR Fettke acknowledged that no patient had lodged a complaint against him. AHPRA acknowledged that no harm came to patients from Fettke's dietary advice, and no significant "risk" was "apparent" as a dietary option.

In September 2018, the Board decided not to take any further regulatory action and cleared Fettke of any breach of Good Medical Practice by referring to its Code of Conduct which states that "good patient care involves encouraging patients to take interest and responsibility for the management of their health and that doctors have a right to inform patients and colleagues of treatments to which they conscientiously object".

Fettke had said he prefers not to amputate the limbs of his patients when simple dietary change can save them. The AHPRA's letter and apology go beyond clearing Fettke professionally but "clearly implies there is no harm in any health professional in Australia recommending LCHF therapies," says Fettke.

Promoting LCHF comes at a price. The current Australian Dietary Guidelines do not promote LCHF. On 30th October 2018, AHPRA dropped all charges against DR Fettke and apologized.

3. *HPCSA VS Prof Timothy Noakes 2014 (210)*Prof Tim Noakes a South African Professor is said to have had a doctor-patient relationship with a breastfeeding mother on Twitter, that information he tweeted was not evidence-based and that it conflicted with South African Dietary Guidelines and that it was dangerous (life-threatening).

The Health Professions Council of South Africa (HPCSA) continued to change tact and goalposts whenever it failed to prove an essential element of its case. He was charged by HPCSA and Association for Dieticians in South Africa (ADSA).

The hearing started in June 2015 and finally reached a conclusion in April 2017. The costs reached into the tens of millions for each party and made headlines as the "Nutrition Trial of the Century".

HPCSA found Prof Noakes innocent of unprofessional conduct on 21st April 2017. The ruling had far-reaching implications for every South African as it gave the seal of approval to the LCHF diet. "We fought the battle for the health of all South Africans," said Noakes. "Now you know the truth that you have been misinformed for 50 years. We all have been and the consequences to our health have been dire".

Conclusion: All the cases have ended up exonerating the Practitioners but all caused significant personal damage to the Doctors concerned.

Very little Nutrition/Dietetics is covered in the curriculum for Medical Students at Undergraduate and Postgraduate levels. Nutritionists/Dieticians are taught and practice mainstream/Conventional Nutrition/Dietetics. The Medical doctors and Nutritionists/Dieticians who have embraced LCHF ketogenic diets had to divert from the mainstream Conventional clinical care due to their personal reasons and or due to frustrations as a result of failure of expected patient treatment outcomes e.g. failure of obese patients to lose weight despite adherence to Conventional Dietary Advice or accidental exposure to LCHF diets clinical trials and effectiveness.

Starting to apply or recommend LCHF diets to patients in a Country or Institution practicing Conventional Medical or Nutritional Guidelines puts one in a collision course with the Government Regulatory Medical Boards, Institutional Administration, fellow Medical Colleagues and other interested parties e.g. "Big Pharma" and processed food industries. No wonder the three most prominent litigations against doctors practicing LCHF diet therapy since 2000 had been instituted by Dietician Boards.

How to avoid malpractice risks when prescribing off-label: Stump: 2008 (211)
"Are physicians liable for Medical Malpractice if an off-label drug they prescribe causes adverse effects? The question was at the heart of a Lawsuit. "The fact that a prescription is off label does not itself increase risk". This case is a detailed example of how to avoid malpractice risks while prescribing off-label.

Though Medical Practitioners prescribing LCHF diets can have action taken against them by patients, Professional bodies, etc. simple steps can reduce the risk of litigation:

a) Informed patient consent: make patients aware of the dietary options, known risks, benefits, short and long term complications, expected outcomes, etc. *LCHF diets can give false positive alcohol breath test. Sudden Unexpected Death in Epilepsy can occur, but it's etiology is not associated with the LCHF diet.*

b) Contra-indications to LCHF diets: congenital metabolic and genetic disorders.

c) Maintain thorough and detailed patient records including Clinical notes on examination, diagnosis, comorbidities, indication for LCHF diet, history of medications e.g. SGLT-2, Dietician/Nutrition reviews, Laboratory tests, daily inpatient and outpatient follow up reviews, etc.

d) Monitor progress and adjust medications, diet etc.

It takes time for Standard Clinical Practice Guidelines to change; it has taken nearly 40 years for American Diabetes Association to incorporate LCHF ketogenic diets as a dietary treatment option for diabetes Type-2.It might take longer for our Government and Diabetes Association to follow suit.

KEY TAKEAWAYS:

- *Prescribing a LCHF diet is within evidence based medicine practiced worldwide.*
- *Simple steps can reduce the risk of litigation. E.g. Detailed patient records.*
- *The practitioner should be aware of the medico legal aspects of the LCHF diet*

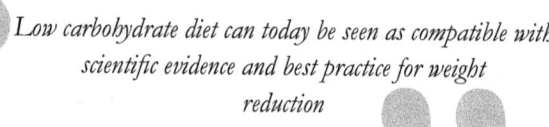

Low carbohydrate diet can today be seen as compatible with scientific evidence and best practice for weight reduction

CHAPTER THIRTY FIVE

ECONOMIC IMPACT OF LCHF KETOGENIC DIET

Non-communicable diseases (NCDs) account for a huge percentage of Worldwide Government expenditure on Health. In Kenya, although the Health Budget has increased by more than 30% (2019 Kenya Budget), it is still short of the 15% target set by African Countries known as Abuja Declaration.

Kenya is undergoing an epidemiological transition marked by a decline in morbidity and mortality due to communicable conditions and an increase in the burden of NCDs which include diseases such as diabetes, hypertension, cancers, cardiovascular diseases, and chronic respiratory diseases.

85% of global deaths due to NCDs are in Low and Middle-Income Countries (LMICs) and the human and economic burdens of NCDs especially in LMICs are not sustainable and are a threat to development.

In Kenya NCDs contribute to over 50% of Inpatient admissions and 40% of hospital deaths, taking a big percentage of the health budget. The prevention strategies would be the most efficient approach in mitigating NCDs in an LMIC like Kenya. An unhealthy diet, physical inactivity, tobacco, and alcohol use are modifiable risk factors.

The results of a study on NCDs in Kenya: "Economic effects and risk factors by Mwai D N University of Nairobi (212) show that low intake of fruit and vegetables, cigarette smoking, alcohol consumption and household income are some of the NCD risk factors.

In **"The rise of non-communicable diseases in Kenya: An examination of the time, and trends and contribution of the changes in diet and physical activity" by Onyango E M et al(213)** showed a rapid rise in the incidence of Circulatory Disease starting in 2001, and of Hypertension and Diabetes starting in 2008.

"In conclusion, the positive correlation between indicators of dietary consumption and physical inactivity and rates of hypertension, circulatory disease and diabetes suggest that the rapid rates in NCDs may be, in part, due to changes in these modifiable factors e.g. rise in per capita GDP and physical inactivity.

Unhealthy diet and physical inactivity, in particular, are associated with obesity, diabetes, cardiovascular disease, and cancer". And these NCDs are associated with chronic inflammation and hyperinsulinemia.

A well-formulated LCHF KD diet is known to lead to weight loss, DMT2 reversal, positively reduce hyperinsulinemia, chronic inflammatory markers, reduce or reverse hypertension, improve lipid profiles and other cardiovascular risk factors.

The WHO recommended *"Best Buy intervention for NCD prevention and Control (2017)"* lists three risk factors and best buy interventions:
a) Tobacco use: raise taxes on tobacco, protect people from tobacco smoke, warn about the dangers of tobacco, and enforce bans on tobacco advertising.
b) Harmful use of alcohol: Raise taxes on alcohol, restrict access to retailed alcohol and enforce bans on alcohol advertising.
c) Unhealthy diet and physical inactivity: Reduce salt intake in food, replace trans fats with polyunsaturated fats, and promote public awareness about the diet and physical inactivity (via mass media).

Kenya needs a more revised 2019 NCDs policy and a revised Diet and Nutrition Policy which reflects the current scientific knowledge and is keeping up with changing Worldwide Dietary Guidelines e.g. there is questionable scientific advantage on the advice to reduce salt intake in food: *PURE STUDY (23)* and, replacing trans-fat with polyunsaturated fat *(26), (36)*.

Changing and implementation of Government Policy and Conventional Guidelines takes time as evidenced by the study by *Pamela A Juma et al "Non-communicable disease prevention policy process in five African countries (214).* This study showed that the Five African countries have the will in implementation of NCD policies but they face implementation gaps".

However, the start of a personal initiative can change the prevalence and prevention of NCDs. *The case of Dr David Unwin in Britain (48), (67)* is a good example. The impact of his LCHF diet primary management of diabetes and obesity has not only transformed the community but has also saved a lot of money for the National Health Service (NHS), the equivalent of our National Hospital Insurance Fund (NHIF).

The Health insurance providers have a lot to gain from *LCHF diet implementation as shown by Dr John Schoonbee (215) a Medical Officer and Senior Health Insurance Manager: InLCHF who benefits financially?* He talks about science and politics in nutrition, the more the mortality of insured people, the more payments. Risk selection and lapses in policy are mainly done by healthy people and mortality rates improve due to the prevention of NCDs.

Life expectancy in USA has decreased due to suicide, drug overdose, diabetes and Metabolic Syndrome. In Sweden LCHF campaigns have decreased diabetes mortality and obesity which is strongly associated with diabetes, cardiovascular disease and cancer.

Diabetes reversal leads to improvement of risk factors e.g. reduced BMI, better lipid profile, fatty liver reversal, the reversal of hyperinsulinemia and hyperglycemia and blood pressure which increase insurance risk; these lead to lower CVD deaths (Stroke and Myocardial Infarction), decreased incidence of cancer and cancer deaths.

The insurance industry is trying to promote the right nutritional advice to reverse diabetes but health insurance firms have to consider liability and reputation and that is why now they can promote LCHF because it has been proven to be safe. Analysis of the life insurance model shows that reversing diabetes will reduce claims by 26% and equally the Government Health Expenditure can be readily reduced with the right nutritional strategy.

Who benefits from the status quo? The Government recommends a diet that contains plenty of starchy foods e.g. rice, bread, potatoes, plenty of fruit and vegetables, some protein-rich foods: meat, fish, beans, poultry, eggs, and milk and dairy products, choosing reduced-fat versions, a little saturated fat, salt and sugar.

The beneficiaries are the people producing and selling the food, the people treating obesity and chronic diseases (drug companies, medical devices, medical doctors, private hospitals, food industry and diet industry, anyone in the longevity risk business, pension funds and annuities).

Who will benefit if the world shifted to LCHF? Certain food segments, State Health Funders (NHS, NHIF,) Life and Health Industry (Insurance Industry) and 7 Billion people on earth.

Bundle protection for each lifestyle: if claims increase then premiums increase but not so fast. Increasing premiums will decrease insurance penetration and increase the already huge protection gap that exists.

Long term data on LCHF diets will enable the Insurance Industry to have long term projections. LCHF diet affordability and the fact that some cultures cannot drop carbs are some of the problems in the implementation of LCHF.

DR David Unwin et al in practical Diabetes 2014; 31 (2) 76-79 (216) shows what could happen to those at risk if they switch and reduce carbohydrates: *"Low carbohydrate diet to achieve weight loss and improve HbA1c in prediabetes and Type-2 diabetes, experience from one General Practitioner:"* This approach is easy to implement in general practice and brings rapid weight loss and improvement in HbA1c.

How could the life insurance industry benefit?
1. Globally change Nutritional Guidelines (consume healthy fat; reduce carbs especially refined sugar/carbs).
2. Change the health of obese and diabetics and related comorbidities.
3. Offer incentives for new and old insurance policyholders who are obese and diabetic to shift to a LCHF diet.
4. LCHF results in less inflammation and chronic diseases, psychiatric, musculoskeletal complaints, reduction in disability claims and an increase in long term protection health claims.

A LCHF diet lifestyle promotes reducing grams of carbs that you consume per day and replacing them with fats. The ketogenic and Atkins diets are types of

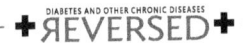

LCHF diets. LCHF diet is an effective way to lose body fat, reduce carbohydrate cravings and overall hunger. It leads to many health benefits: reverses DMT2, treats neurological diseases (epilepsy, Alzheimer's diseases), reduces body fat, lowers/normalizes high blood pressure, reduces inflammation related to heart disease, and chronic pain syndrome-like arthritis, augments cancer therapy etc.

LCHF diet encourages eating real food: eggs, oils (coconut, avocado, olive), fish, meat and poultry, full dairy milk and dairy products, non-starchy vegetables, nuts/seeds, and spices and discourages eating of starches, sugar and sugary drinks, sweeteners, starchy vegetables, and processed foods.

LCHF diet is sustainable, benefits the patient, Country, Government, Health Insurance firms but not the BIG PHARMA and processed food/sweet beverages companies!"

KEY TAKEAWAYS:

- *85% of global deaths are due to non-communicable diseases (NCD's)*
- *The beneficial economic impact of the LCHF diet can be felt by government agencies, health insurance agencies and individuals.*
- *The LCHF diet is an important tool for the prevention, treatment and reversal of noncommunicable diseases.*

"An unhealthy diet, physical inactivity, tobacco, and alcohol use are modifiable risk factors.

CHAPTER THIRTY SIX

THE FUTURE OF KETOGENIC DIETS

*I*s *LCHF ketogenic diet a fad?* A Fad is an intense and widely shared enthusiasm for something, especially one that is short-lived and without basis in the object's qualities; a craze.

Keto and fasting: latest fad or the keys to optimum health: Jimmy Moore(217)
"He gives the definition of fad, history of the Banting diet (the letter opulence) in 1863 which was the recommended diet for diabetes and obesity until Ancel Keys introduced his fat Heart Hypothesis in 1959 to the modern use of low fat high carb diets. Ketones were discovered in 1921 in patients who were on a fast mimicking diet.

Ketogenic diet use was affected by the discovery of antiepileptic drugs and the recommendation of low fat high carb diet and the blaming of fat not sugar for obesity and disease leading to 1977 American Guidelines which have been blamed for the obesity epidemic. Chronic inflammation is mainly caused by sugar and vegetable oils and is associated with major non-communicable diseases.

Fasting is not treatment for illness but treatment for wellness. Spiritual fasting is encouraged. From Hippocrates to Plato, therapeutic fasting continued through the ages to 1980 when low-fat high-carb diets were introduced and fasting was forgotten. But in 2016 Yoshimori Ohsumi won a Nobel Prize on autophagy and fasting. DR Jason Fung and others have since contributed to the present upsurge in application of therapeutic fasting.

Prior to 400BC, Epilepsy was presumed to be a disease caused by supernatural forces; but about that year a text known as the Hippocratic corpus: on the sacred disease challenged that view, suggesting that dietary fasting may provide relief from seizures.

William Banting in 1863 recommended a low carbohydrate high fat diet which was taught in medical schools for weight loss and health up to 1959.

A discovery by Rollin Woodyatt in 1921 determined that when the liver is starved of carbohydrate it releases three components; *beta*-hydroxybutyrate, aceto-acetate, and acetone. Today they are classified as ketone bodies.

Russel Wilder from Mayo Clinic coined the word ketogenic diet due to the high levels of ketones generated from a low carbohydrate diet.

Epilepsy could be treated not through fasting but fasting from carbohydrates while consuming high quality fats and other nutrients i.e. Ketogenic diets became the substitute for fasting.

In the 1940s anticonvulsant medications were discovered and for decades they surpassed ketogenic diets as the preferred treatment for Epilepsy.

Then DR Ancel Keys came with his fat heart hypothesis and dietary advice leading to present-day high carbohydrate low-fat recommendations for the prevention of heart disease. Blame for heart disease was shifted from sugar to fat.

In the 1977 Food Pyramid, saturated fats were blamed for heart disease. The rate of obesity and heart disease went up in the USA. Then Atkins diet was introduced in 1972 followed by more research on applications of ketogenic diets and modified Atkins diet.

A decade of modified Atkins Diet: 2003-2013, results, insights and future directions: Eric Kossoff et al (218) the modified Atkins diet (MAD) has been used since 2003 for the treatment of children and adults with refractory epilepsy. This alternative ketogenic diet is started in Clinic without fasting, hospitalization and restriction of proteins, calories or fluid intake. After 10 years of continued use about 400 patients had been reported in over 30 studies of the MAD as a treatment for intractable seizures, with results demonstrating similar efficacy to the ketogenic diet and improved tolerability.

The MAD is being increasingly used in the adult population. Clinical trials have provided insight into the mechanisms of action of dietary therapies overall. This review discusses the past decade's action of experience with MAD as well as predictions for its role in the treatment of epilepsy a decade from then.

The ketogenic diet and its role in children with refractory epilepsy were revisited in 1997: *The ketogenic diet revisited: Back to the future: Douglas R Nordli et al (219)* "He revisited the use of ketogenic diet (KD) in 1997 and whether it deserved a prominent role in the management of pediatric refractory epilepsy.

In 1994, a high profile case of epilepsy successfully controlled using the ketogenic diet returned the ketogenic diet to the Modern era. In 1977, Meryl Streep starred about the diet in the film "First do no Harm"when debilitating conventional treatments fail, a woman tries a controversial diet for her epileptic son (Seth Adkins).

The Ketogenic diet did not disappear after BIG-Food and BIG-Pharma ostracized it.

Ketogenic diet is reinvented from medical to fitness diet; for models to Marshall Fighters, to unstoppable trend as a potential cure for cancer etc".

Sustainability and future of LCHF ketogenic diet is discussed in many clinical reviews (169), (170), (171), (172), (173), (174).

Modifying the ketogenic diet to a more flexible modified Atkins diet (MAD) may enable easy sustainability while maintaining its effectiveness. The ketogenic diet is preferable for children less than 2 years while MAD is a better option in adolescents and adults in management of epilepsy and other conditions where ketogenic diet is indicated

Ketogenic diets: Boon or Bane: J Skilpa (220) "Ketogenic diets are now being used for obesity. Physiological principles of ketogenic diets, benefits, adverse effects, different types of ketogenic diets and its sustainability are discussed in this review. The future of LCHF ketogenic diet is bright.

Mozaffarian D Daruish et al: The US 2015 dietary guidelines ending the 35% limit for total dietary fat: (221) and also dropped dietary cholesterol as a "nutrient of concern".

The recent *"American Diabetic Association (ADA) and European Association for the Study of Diabetes approval of low carb diet for the management of diabetes type-2 in adults October 2018" (54) and the ADA consensus statement 2019* point to a paradigm shift from High Carb Low Fat towards recognition of the clinical role of a Low carb High Fat (LCHF) ketogenic diets.

Ketogenic diet market analysis is projected to witness rapid growth by forecast to 2023. *Ketogenic diet Market report forecast 2018-2023: Market research Future July 2019: (222)* "Ketogenic diet a low carb high fat and moderate protein plays a role in improving Insulin resistance and management of chronic diseases. Elevation in the level of consumer awareness regarding the health benefits aligned with the ketogenic diet is driving the market majorly. The emergence of ketogenic diet "keto" certification reflects positively on the growth of KD market.

North America (first) and Europe (second) accounts for the most significant share of the global ketogenic diet Market.

KEY TAKEAWAYS:

- *Fasting is not a treatment for illness but a treatment for wellness.*
- *The LCHF diet is not a fad, it has been used throughout human history.*
- *The LCHF diet is sustainable and its renewed clinical role is being officially approved worldwide.*
- *The future of the LCHF diet is bright.*

"It's easier to fool people than to convince them that they have been fooled"
Mark Twain.

"When diet is wrong, medicine is of no use. When diet is correct, medicine is of no need."
- Ancient Aryuvedic Proverb

REFERENCES: BOOKS, JOURNALS, CONFERENCE LECTURES

1. Michael Gelfand,
   1948
   "The Sick African"

2. Rita Lakhtakia:
   Aug 2013
   "The history of diabetes mellitus"
   Sultan Qaboos University Medical Journal
   (3)368-370

3. Allan F L:
   1972
   "Diabetes before and after insulin"
   (16) Med. Hist.
   266-73

4. DR Chukwuemeka Nwanesi:
   2015
   "Diabetes Mellitus"
   A complete ancient and modern historical perspective
   Webried Central Article
   6 (2)

5. Bell G: et al: 1980
   "Sequence of human insulin gene"
   Nature
   284-32

6. Mayo clinic.com
   "Pancreatic Transplantation"

7. Adapted from DF: Diabetes Atlas 2015

8. Sarah Hallberg
   Reversing Type-2 Diabetes starts with ignoring the guidelines

9. DR Eric Westman
   "Treatment of Diabetes"

10. DR Jason Fung
    "Insulin toxicity and to cure Type-2 Diabetes"

11. Prof Jeff Volek
    "The art and science of Low Carbohydrates living"

12. William Yancy, Marjorie Foy and Eric Westman
    (2005)
    "A Low Carbohydrate Ketogenic diet to treat Type-2 Diabetes"
    Nutrition and Metabolism
    2, 34

13. Carole David and Atta Saltos
    "American Dietary Recommendations"

14. Julia Reedy:
    2016
    "How the US Low Fat Diet Recommendations of 1977 contributed to the declining Health of Americans "

15. David Diamond:
"Demonization and Deception on saturated fat,
Cholesterol and Heart Disease."

16. Hussein Dashti et al: 2016
Long Term Effects of Ketogenic diet in obese subjects with high cholesterol Level:
Mol. Cell. Biochem.

17. Richard Feinman et al
Jan, 2015
"Dietary carbohydrate as the first approach to Diabetes Management: a Critical Review and Evidence base.
Nutrition Vol. 31: issue 1; 1-13

18. Jack Wolfson
"The truth about cholesterol

19. DR Peter Attia
"Readdressing dietary guidelines"

20. DR Jonny Bowden
"The Great Cholesterol Myth"

21. Nina Teicholz
"The US Dietary Guidelines and scientific evidence"

22. DR Tim Noakes
"Challenging conventional dietary advice/guidelines, the brief story behind the writing of LORE NUTRITION"

23. DR Andrew Mente
"Diet and Cardiovascular disease; Message from PURE STUDY"

24. Zoe Harcombe
"Nutritional nuggets to combat conventional dietary advice/guidelines: Challenging beliefs"

25. Nina Teicholz
"Vegetable Oils: The unknown story"

26. Nina Teicholz
Vegetable Oils:
"The untold story and the dietary guidelines"

27. DR David Diamond
"Dietary sense and nonsense in the war on saturated fat"

28. DR Aseem Malhotra
"Too much medicine and great statin con"

29. DR Maryanne Demasi
Jan 2018
"Statin wars; have we been misled by evidence?"
Br. J Sports Medicine

30. "International Table of glycemic index and glycemic load control values"
2012

31. Rabecca A. Abere et al
2007
"Glycemic index of cassava and sweet potatoes consumed in Western Kenya"
Food Science and quality management
Vol. 63

32. Rabecca A. Abere et al
2007
"Glycemic index of cassava and sweet potatoes consumed in Western Kenya"
Food Science and quality management
Vol. 63

33. Waudo et al
2017
"An investigation on glycemic index of local foods and dietetics. Management of diabetes mellitus: A study in Kisii and Homa Bay District Hospital"
Kenyatta University Dept. of Foods, Nutrition and dietetics.

34. Smith G. Nthata et al
2018
"Fermentation and germination improve nutritional value of cereals and legumes through activation of endogenous enzymes"
Food Science and Nutrition
6(8)
2446-2468

35. "Kenya Medical guidelines for the management of Diabetes"
2nd Edition 2018

36. DR Paul Mason
"Saturated Fat is not dangerous"

37. A/Prof Ken Sikaris
"Cholesterol: when to worry".

38. DR Stephen Phinney
"The art and science of nutritional Ketosis"

39. DR Richard Feinman PhD
Ketogenic diets and Diabetes
January 2015

40. DR Eric Westman: LCHF and Diabetes:
"Theory and Clinical experience"

41. Mike Mutzel
"Fasting, Autophagy and Exercise"

42. DR Jason Fung
"Application of intermittent fasting in medicine"

43. Prof Roy Taylor
"Reversing the irreversible: Type-2 Diabetes and you;
Journal of endocrinological investigation June 2019
"Freedom from Diabetes"
Lancet 2017

44. Paoli A: 2013
"Beyond weight Loss: A review of therapeutic uses of very low carbohydrates (ketogenic) diet:"
European journal of Clinical Nutrition
67; 788-796

45. DR Dominic D'Agostino:
"Emerging applications of the Ketogenic diet"

46. Prof Tim Noakes
"Real Meal Revolution"

47. DR David Unwin
"The glycemic index helping patients in primary care"

48. DR Amy Mackenzie PHD
"Literature Review: The evidence of low carbohydrates nutrition for Diabetics.
VIRTA HEALTH

49. Sami T Azar et al:
2016:
"Benefits of Ketogenic diet for management of Type-2 Diabetes: A review"
Obesity and Eating disorders
Vol. 2; 2-22

50. Mobbs C V et al:
May 16 2013:
"Treatment of Diabetes and Diabetic complications with a Ketogenic diet"
Journal of Child Neurology.

51. Mark Cucurella et al:
2019
"A Clinician's guide to low carbohydrate diet for remission of DMT2; towards a standard care protocol"
Diabetes management
Vol. 9, issue 1

52. 'Dietary carbohydrate is not an essential nutrient: Institute of Medicine US. Dietary reference for energy carbohydrate, fiber, fatty acids cholesterol, protein and amino acids."
2005:
Washington DC. The National Academic Press

53. DR Eric Westman
May 2002
'" Dietary carbohydrates is not an essential nutrient: Is dietary carbohydrate essential for human nutrition"
The American Journal of Clinical Nutrition
Vol. 75 issue 5; 951-953

54. October 2018:
"American Diabetes Association (ADA): "
Nutrition Guidelines.

55. Belinda S Lennerz et al
"Management of type-1 Diabetes with a very low carbohydrate diet"
Pediatrics Vol. 141 No. 6

56. DR Troy Stapleton
"Carbohydrate restriction in Diabetes Management".

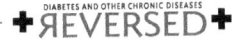

57. Jessica L Turton:2018
"Low Carbohydrate for Type-1 Diabetes Mellitus: A systematic review"
PLos one: 13 (3)

58. Keich R Runyan MD
"Management of Type-1 Diabetes with a ketogenic diet"

59. Ail J Ahola et al: 2019
Carbohydrate intake and cardiometabolic risk factors in type-1 diabetes
Diabetes Research and Clinical Practice

60. DR Richard Bernstein:
DR Bernstein Diabetes Solution Book.

61. DR Olivia Rimmington:
Low Carb Nutrition for T1DM

62. Sam Scott
2019
"Carbohydrate restriction in Type-1 Diabetes: A realistic therapy for improved glycemic control and athletes performance"
Nutrients 11. 1022.

63. Paolo P
2018,
Latent Autoimmune Diabetes in Adults: Current Status and new Horizons.
Endocrinol.Metab. (Seoul) Jun. 33 (3); 147-159.

64. Cameron F J et al:
1997
"Maturity onset Diabetes of the Young (MODY): Three cases report and new perspective"
J. Pediatri. Endocrinol.Metab.Jan-Feb.

65. Maturity Onset Diabetes Of the Young (MODY):
Health Topics
Harvard Health Publishing: April 2019. October 2018:
"American Diabetes Association (ADA): "
Nutrition Guidelines.

66. Agarwal et al
2002
"Maturity Onset Diabetes of the Young"
JIACM; 3 (3); 271-277.

67. DR David Unwin
2019
Substantial and sustained improvements in blood, weight, and liquid profiles from a carbohydrate restricted diet: An observational study of Insulin resistant patients in primary care:
International journal of environmental research and Public Health

68. Hallberg S.I et al
    Dhanpuri et al
    Diabetic Therapy 2018
    9 (2) 583-612
    "Effective and safety of a novel care needed for the management of DMT2 at one year. An open label, non-randomized controlled study"
    European journal of Clinical Nutrition
    Cardiovascular diabetal
    2018, 17-56

69. DR Eric Westman
    "Ketogenic way of eating for lymph disorders"

70. Leslyn Keith
    "Diet and lifestyle for lymphatic disorders; Implementing a ketogenic diet"

71. Neil et al
    June 2014
    "Ketogenic diet in adolescents and adults with Epilepsy"
    Seizure
    23 (6) 439-42

72. Payne N E et al:2014
    "The ketogenic related diets in adolescents and adults: A review"
    Epilepsia 2011, 52 (11) 1941-8.

73. DR Eric Kossoff:
    "Ketogenic diet for Epilepsy: a century of progress

74. Tanya J William et al
    2017
    "The role of ketogenic diet"
    Clinical neurophysiological practice.
    154-160

75. Alexandria Brambilia et al
    2014
    "Improvement of cardiomyopathy after high fat diet in two siblings with glycogen storage disease Type 3"
    JIMD; 17, 91-95.

76. Aubert G et al: 2016
    The failing heart relies on ketone bodies as a fuel
    Circulation: 133 (8) 698-705

77. Sathya Krishnasamy et al
    July 2018
    "Diabetic Gastroparesis: Principles and current trends in management"
    Diabetes Therapy
    9 (Supp) 1-42

78. Gupta L.
    "Ketogenic diets in endocrine disorders current perspective: Journal of Postgraduate medicine"
    October 2017
    Page 242-251.

79. Dyer et al: 2018
"Ketogenic diet in group 1 pulmonary Hypertension patient:
Am. J Respir, Crit. Care Med.
197-A3712

80. Susan Masino et al Trinity College USA
2013
'Ketogenic diets and pain"
J. Child. Neurol.

81. DR Peter Brukner
"Inflammation"

82. DR Doron Sher
"Arthritis and weight loss: A case study "

83. DR Sioban Huggins
"Investigating Inflammation"

84. Dr Evelyne Bourdua-Roy and Dr Hala Lahlou
"Can LCHF and ketogenic diet improve chronic pain?"

85. Shweta Khanna et al
2017
"Managing Rheumatoid Arthritis with Dietary interventions"
Frontiers in Nutrition
4:52

86. Elizabeth M. Masko et al
2010
"Low carbohydrate diet and prostate cancer: How low is low enough?"
Cancer prevention research (Philadelphia P.a)

87. Jocelyn Tan Shalaby MD
Feb. 2017
"Ketogenic diets and cancer emerging evidence"
Fed.Pract.
34 (supp. 1)

88. John Mavropoulos et al
2006
"Is there a role for a low carbohydrate ketogenic diet in the management of prostate cancer?"
Urology
68 (1), 15-18

89. DR Adrianne Scheck
"Tumor metabolism and the ketogenic diet"

90. Dr Colin Champ
"Dietary recommendations for cancer, Warburg Metabolism: Clinical applications"

91. DR Thomas N. Seyfield PHD
"Cancer: Metabolism disease with metabolic solutions"

92. Prof. Angela Poff:
'Ketogenic diet, cancer metabolism and the Warburg effects"

93. Prof Angela Poff
"Exploiting cancer metabolism with ketosis and hyperbaric oxygen"

94. DR Dawn Lemmane
'Carbohydrate restrictions to enhance cancer therapy"

95. Bostock et al
March 2017
"Current status of the ketogenic diet in psychiatry"
Frontiers in Psychiatry
8 (43)

96. Dr Georgia Ede
June 30 :2017
'How ketogenic diet helps in psychiatric disorders; A new 2017 review"
PsychologyToday

97. Dr Georgia Ede
March 27 :2018
'Ketogenic diets and psychiatric medications"
PsychologyToday

98. Brutzke E. et al
2018
"Ketogenic diet as a metabolic therapy for mood disorders; Evidence and developments"
Neurosci: Biobehav Rev.

99. James R Phelps et al:
2013
"The ketogenic diet for type-2 Bipolar Disorder" (Neurocase)
The Neural Basis of Cognition, Vol. 19 issue 5.

100. DR Georgia Ede
Brain needs meat:
Mental benefits of the carnivorous diet

101. Hussein Dashti et al
2004
"Long term effects of a ketogenic diet in obese patients"
Experimental and clinical cardiology
9(3) 200-2005

102. DR Lucy Burns:
"The Hormonal Approach to Obesity"

103. Divicolantonio et al:
July 2018:
"Sugar Addiction, is it Real?"
Brit. Journ. Sports Medicine:
52 (14), 910-913

104. Westwater M L et al:
Nov. 2016
"Sugar addiction: State of the Science "
European J. of Nutrition
55; (Supp 2)

105. Dr Eric Westman, William Yancy et al:
2018
"Use of a low carbohydrate ketogenic diet to treat obesity"
Primary care Reports
Issue Oct

106. Wajeed Masood
2019
"Ketogenic diet: Review article
PubMed March 1019

107. Clifton M. Peter
2008
Dietary treatment of obesity
Nat. Clin. Pract.Gastroenterol.Hepatol.
5 (12); 672-681

108. Stephen Cunanne:
"Can ketones slow down Alzheimer's disease?"

109. DR Mary Newport
'Unconventional but effective therapy for Alzheimer's treatment"

110. Amy Berger
2018
"Alzheimer's disease Type 3 Diabetes"
KETOCON

111. Klaus W. Lange
Katherine M .Lange et al
November 2016
"Ketogenic diets and Alzheimer's disease"
Research Gate

112. Dariusz Włodarek
Jan 2019
"Role of ketogenic diets in neurodegenerative disease (Alzheimer's, Parkinson's disease)"
Nutrients
11(1): 169

113. Marta Rusek et al
2019
Ketogenic diet in Alzheimer's disease: Review
Int. J, Mol. Sci.

114. Sheyda Shaafi et al
Dec 4 2014
"Ketogenic diet provides neuro protective effects against asthmic stroke neuronal damages"
Advanced pharmaceutical bulletin
Supp 2: 479-481

115. Jack Woodfield: Sept. 2017
"Inflammation after stroke or traumatic brain injury"
Nature Communication Journal TUE. 26.

116. Poplawski et al
2011
"Reversal of Diabetic Nephropathy by a ketogenic diet' PLos: one: e 18604

117. Mark Y. Z. Wong
2018
"Dietary intake and diabetic retinopathy: A Systematic Review"
PLos One 13(1)

118. Dr Stephen Phinney and Virta Team
"Can I reverse diabetic nephropathy or retinopathy with a ketogenic diet?"

119. Trotta M C et al: 2019
The activation of retinol HCA2 receptors by systemic beta hydroxybutyrate inhibits diabetic retinol damage through reduction of endoplasmic reticulum stress and NLRP3 inflammasome.
PLos One

120. O Shen MD
2000
"Diabetic gastropathy: A practical approach to a vexing problem"
Cleveland Clinic. Journal of Medicine
Vol 67(9)

121. Brooke Barley PHD , Stephen Phinney PH D and Jeff Volek PHD
January 15: 2019
"Polycystic ovarian syndrome, insulin resistance and inflammation"
Virta Health

122. Mavropoulos I.C. et al:
2005
"The effects of low carbohydrate ketogenic diet on the polycystic ovary syndrome: A pilot study"
Nutri.Meta.(Lond.)
2: 35

123. Neal et al: 2008
"Ketogenic diet for the treatment of childhood epilepsy: A randomized controlled trial.
Lancet Neurol. Vol. 7, issue 6, 500-506

124. Keene DL et al: 2006
"A systematic review of the use of the ketogenic diet in childhood epilepsy disease: A review article"
Pediatric Neural

125. Martin K et al
2012
"Ketogenic diet and other dietary treatments of epilepsy: Review article: Cochrane Database"

126. Antonio Paoli et al: 2014
"Ketogenic diet in neuromuscular and neurodegenerative diseases"
Biomed Research International: Vol.2014

127. Thomas Seyfield
"Ketone Strong: Emerging evidence for a therapeutic role of ketone bodies in the neurological and neurodegenerative diseases"

128. Macdonald T.J. et al: 2018
"Ketogenic diet for adult neurological disorders: Review article
Neurotherapeutics: Vol. 15 issue 4 1018-1031

129. Macdougale A et al: 2018
"Ketogenic diet as a treatment of traumatic brain injury: A scoping review"
Brain Injury
Vol. 32, 2018 issue 4: 416-422

130. Erdman et al: 2011
"Nutrition and Traumatic Brain Injury: Improving acute and sub-acute health outcomes in military personnel"
National Academy of Sciences

131. Barbanti P. et al: 2017
"Ketogenic diet migraine Rationale, findings and Perspective"
Neurol. Sci.; Vol.38 suppl. 1ppg 111-115

132. A/Prof Ken Sikaris
'Fatty Liver and Chemical Pathology"

133. DR Stephen Phinney
"Ketogenic diets and endurances: performance still controversial after four decades"

134. Prof. Jeff Volek
"Physical performance and ketogenic diets"

135. Richard A La Fountain et al 2019
"Extended ketogenic diet and physical training intervention in military personnel"
Military Medicine: D01:10:1093

136. Brianna MacDaniel et al
"Ketones, Ketogenic diets and the Skin"
Skin J. 2 (1); 18-19

137. Antonio Paoli et al
Feb. 2012
Nutrition and acne: Therapeutic potential of ketogenic diets"
Skin Pharm. and Physiol.;25: 111-117
25 (3) 111-7

138. Matt Titlow
Monday February 2017
"The definite guide to Macronutrients in the ketogenic diet"
Compound solutions.

139. DR Loren Cordain PHD
March 2018
"Ketogenic diet long term Nutritional and Metabolic deficiencies"
Research Gate.

140. Forsythie C.E., Stephen Phinney et al: 2008
"A comparison of low fat and low carbohydrate diets on circulating fatty acid composition and markers of inflammation "
Lipids (2008); 43: 65-77

141. Brianna Stubbs PHD
Reduce inflammation: Why ketogenic diet and exogenous ketones are key: Research round up"

142. Yun Hee Youm et al
2015
"Ketone body beta hydroxybutyrate blocks the NLRP3; Inflammasome mediated in inflammatory disease."
Nat. med: 21 (3) 263-269

143. Susan A Masino PH D Oxford University Press
"Ketogenic diet and metabolic therapies: expanded roles in Health and disease"

144. DR Gary Fettke
"Nutrition and Inflammation"
145. IDF School of Diabetes"

146. Moira Lawler
2019
"Diet and Nutrition review"
8:27

147. Furmli S. et al
Oct 9 2018
"Therapeutic use of intermittent fasting for people with Type-2
diabetes as an alternative to insulin"
BMJ Case Rep.

148. Mattson M.P. et al
2016
"Impact on intermittent fasting on Health and disease processes: Aging Research Reviews"
(39) 46-58

149. Harris L. et al
2018
"Intermittent fasting intervention for treatment of overweight and obesity in adults: A systematic review and med. Analysis"
JB database of systematic reviews and implementation reports
16(1) 507-547

150. Anton S. D et al
2018
"Flipping the metabolic switch: understanding and applying the Health benefits of fasting"
Obesity 26: (2) 254-268

151. Horre B.D. et al
2015
"Health benefits of intermittent fasting: Hormesis or Harm?
A systematic review."
American journal of clin. Med. 102 (2) 464-70

152. DR Robert Szabo
"Introduction to therapeutic fasting

153. Gnanou J et al:
2015
Effects of Ramadhan fasting on glucose and homeostasis and adiponectin levels on healthy adult males"
J. Diabetes Metab. Disord.
Vol. 14:55

154. Mehanna H M et al
2008
Refeeding syndrome: What is it and how to treat and prevent it:
BMJ: 336, 1405-1498

155. DR   Jason Fung and Jimmy Moore
'Why you should not fear fasting"

156. Brandhorst S; Longo V D
Dietary restrictions and nutrition in the prevention and treatment of cardiovascular disease"
Circulation Research: Aha Journals.Org.

157. Escober et al
Nov. 2018
"Autophagy and aging maintaining the proteome through exercise and caloric restriction"
Aging cell vol. 18 issue 1(1)

158. DR Paul Mason
Update 2019
"High Cholesterol on a ketogenic (plus do statins work)?

159. Uffer Ravnskov et al
2016
"Lack of an association or an inverse association between low density – lipoprotein cholesterol and mortality in the elderly: A   systematic review"
BMJ open Vol 6 issue 6

160. DR Phinney and Dr Mackenzie
"How does Virta treatment affects Heart Health and Cardiovascular disease?"

161. DR Sarah Hallberg MD
"Ketogenic diet and heart disease"

162. Kosinski et al: May 2017

"Effects of ketogenic diets on cardiovascular risk factors: Evidence from animal and human studies:"

Nutrients 9, 517

163. Uffer Ravnskov et al

2018

LDL-C does not cause cardiovascular disease; A comprehensive review of the current literature"

Expert review of Clinical Pharmacology

Vol 11 issue 10

164. Brett Scher

"Low Carb/High Fat and Heart"

165. A/Prof Ken Sikaris

"HBA1c, Insulin and Cardiovascular risk"

166. A/Prof Ken Sikaris

"Blood tests to assess your Cardiovascular risk"

167. DR Eric Thorn

"Is keto bad for your Heart?"

168. "American Diabetes Association"

1986 July

Diabetes Care

9(4) 434

169. Mariko Sanada et al

2018

"Efficiency of a moderately low carbohydrates diet in a 36 months observational study of Japanese patients with Type-2 diabetes"

Nutrients

Vol. 10(5), 528

170. Carole Freeman:

"Keto sustainability"

171. Peter Ballerstedt:

"Ruminant reality" KETOCON 2018

172. Nicole Moore:

"LCHF Challenges"

173. DR Andreas Eenfeldt:

"Maintaining weight loss and Type-2 Reversal"

174. Nina Teicholz:

"Red meat and Health"

175. Rashmi Sinha et al:

2009

"Meat intake and Mortality: A prospective study of over half a million people":

Arch. Intern. Med. March 23; 169 (6): 562-571

176. "The European Food and Safety Authority: Nitrate in vegetables, scientific opinion on the panel of contaminants of food chain".
EFSA Journal, 2008, 689, 1-79

177. Dafna Sussman et al:
May 2013:
Effects of a ketogenic diet during pregnancy on embryonic growth in the mouse:
BMC Pregnancy and Childbirth 13 (1); 109

178. Lily Nichols:
Real food for Pregnancy: The Science and Wisdom of optimal Prenatal Nutrition.

179. Lily Nichols:
"Real Food for Gestational Diabetes".

180. Lily Nichols:
Is Low Carb High Fat Safe during Pregnancy?

181. Sadurskis A et al:1988
"Energy Metabolism, Body Composition and milk production in healthy Swedish Women during Lactation"
AM; J. Clin.Nutri.49; 259-65.

182. Panel on micronutrients etc.
Institute of Medicine; National Academic Press.

183. Williamson D F et al
1994
"A Prospective Study of Childbearing and 10 year old gain in US white Women"
Int. Journal of obesity and related metabolic disorders
18 (8) 561-569

184. Wolfe W S S et al:
1997
"Parity associated Body Weight: Modification by socio-demographic and behavioral factors"
Obs. Res. 5: 131-41

185. Mahamoud Mohammed et al:
2009
"Effects of dietary macronutrient composition under modern hypocaloric intake on maternal adaptation during lactation"
The American journal of clinical nutrition
Vol. 89, issue 6; 1821-27.

186. Park Y et al:
1999
"High fat dietary product consumption increases rumeric and total lipid concentration in human milk"
Lipids: 34; 543-9.

187. Butte N F et al:
1984:
"The effect of maternal diet and body composition on lactational performance"
Am. J. Clin. Nutri. 39; 296-306.

188. Dusdieker L B et al:
1994:
Is milk production impaired by dieting during lactation?"
Am. J. Clin. Nutri.59, 833-40.

189. Brair F et al
2016
"Impact of maternal nutrition on breast milk composition: A systematic Review"
Am. J. Clin. Nutri.104 (3); 646-62.

190. Brewer M M
1989
Postpartum changes in maternal weight and body fat deposits in lactating v/s nonlactating women
Am. J. Clin. Nutri. 49, 259-65

191. Lovelady C A et al
2000
The effect of weight loss in overweight lactating women on the growth of their infants"
N. Engl. J. Med.; 342, 449-53.

192. Innis S M et al
2014

Impact of maternal diet on human milk composition and neurological development of infants: Review article.
Am. J. Clin. Nutri.99, (3); 734-41

193. Barrela C et al
Jan 2018
Impact of Maternal diet during pregnancy and lactation on the fatty acid composition of erythrocytes and breast milk of Chilean Women.
Nutrients 28; 10 (7), 839

194. Marangoni Franca et al
2016
Maternal diet and nutrient requirements in Pregnancy and breastfeeding: An Italian Consensus Document.
Nutrients: Oct 8 (10); 629

195. Craig A Johnson et al
2013
The role of low calorie sweeteners in Diabetes
Eur. Endocrinol. 9 (2) 96-98

196. DR Doron Sher:
Artificial sweeteners

197. Ignatio Valencia et al
2002
"General Anesthesia and the ketogenic diet: Clinical experience in nine patients"
Epilepsia
43(5)525 -529

198. Ichikawa et al,
2006
"Anesthetic management of a pediatric patient on a ketogenic diet"
J. Anesth.
20(2) 135-7

199. Hinton et al
1982
"Diet induced ketosis in epilepsy and anesthesia metabolic changes in three patients on a ketogenic diet"
Anaesthesia; Vol 37, 39-42

200. Baumeister F. A. et al
2004
"Fatal propofol infusion syndrome in association with ketogenic diet"
Neuro paediatrics

201. Saito J. et al
2011
"General Anaesthesia with propofol for a pediatric patient on ketogenic diet:" Masui.

202. James Mcneely MD
2008
"Perioperative management of a pediatric patient on the ketogenic diet"
Pediatric Anesthesia
10(1) 103-106

203. Soysal et al
2016
"Pediatric patients on Ketogenic diets undergoing General Anesthesia: A medical review."
J. Clinical Anesth,
170-175

204. Leonett F et al
2015
"Very low carbohydrate ketogenic diet before Bariatric surgery; Prospective evaluation of a sequential diet"
Obes.Surg.

205. Hurwitz
Oct. 30 2004
"How does evidence based guidance influence determination of medical negligence?"
BMJ

206. Brunner L.H et al
2012
"Beyond the standard care: A new model to judge medical negligence"
Clin.Orthop.Relat.Res.

207. Piennar
2011
"An analysis of evidence-based medicine in contest of medical negligence litigation"

208. 2007 NBHW v/s Annika Dahlqvist (prescribing)LCHF for T2D/obese patients)

209. AHPRA v/s Gary Fette (Lack of qualification to advise patients on nutrition" 2014

210. HPCSA (2017) v/s Tim Noakes

211. Stump
Oct. 2008
"How to avoid malpractice risks when prescribing off label."
Neurology Today p (20) 25-26

212. Mwai D N
2019
Non-communicable diseases in Kenya: Economic effects and risk Factors
University of Nairobi (CHSS)

213. Onyango E.M.
2018
"An examination of the time and trends and contribution of the changes in diet and physical activity"
Journal of Epidemiology and Global Health. Vol 8 issue 1-2

214. Pamela A Juma et al
2018
"Non-communicable disease prevention policy process in five African countries"
BMC Public Health 18: 961

215. Dr John Schoonbee
"LCHF; Who benefits financially"

216. DR David Unwin et al
2014
Low carbohydrate diet to achieve weight loss and improve HBA1c in diabetes and prediabetes: Experience from one general practice
Practical Diabetes 31 (2); 76-79

217. Jimmy Moore
Keto and fasting; latest Fad or the key to Optimal Health?

218. Eric Kossof et al:
2013
A decade of modified Atkins diet: 2003-2013: Results, insights and future directions.
Epilepsy and behavior.

219. Douglas K. Nordli et al
1997
"Ketogenic revisited book to the future"
Epilepsia 8 (7) 743-749

220. J. Skilpa
2018 Sept. 20
"Ketogenic Diets Doon or Bane"
The Indian journal of Medical Research
1; 148 (3) 251-253

221. Mozaffarian D Daruish et al
2015
The Us Dietary Guidelines and the 35% limit for total dietary fat
JAMA; 313 (24)

222. July 26 2019
"Ketogenic Diet Market Report Forecast: 2018-2023

ABBREVIATIONS

AHPRA	Australian Health Practitioner Regulation Agency
ANTI GAD	Anti Glutamine acid Decarboxylase
ADHD	Attention Deficit Hyperactivity Disorder
ADSA	Association of Dieticians in South Africa
AD	Alzheimer's disease
ALS	Amyotrophic Lateral Sclerosis
ALT	Alanine Aminotransferase Test
ASD	Autism Spectrum Disorders
AST	Aspartate Transaminase
ASCVD	Atherosclerotic Cardiovascular Disease
AGES	Advanced Glycation End Products
APO-A	Lipoprotein – A
APO-B	Lipoprotein –B
ARR	Absolute Risk Reduction
ADR	American Dietary Recommendations
ADA	American Diabetes Association
AHA	American Heart Association
ARA	Arachidonic Acid
ATP	Adenosine Triphosphate
BRAF VLODE	Gene mutation
BDNF	Brain Derived Neurotrophic Factor
BSL	Blood Sugar Level
BPH	Benign Prostatic Hypertrophy
BP	Blood Pressure
BMI	Body Mass Index

BHB	Beta Hydroxybutyrate
C-Peptide	Insulin Production by Product
CT SCAN	computerized Tomography
CAC Score	Coronary Artery Calcium Score
CIMT	Carotid Intima Media Thickness
CML	Chronic Myeloid Leukemia
CRP	C - reactive protein
COQ10	Coenzyme Q10
CNS	Central Nervous System
CO	Carbon Monoxide
Carb	Carbohydrate
CHD	Coronary Heart Disease
CVD	Cardiovascular Disease
DAA	Dietician Association of Australia
DCD	Developmental Coordination Disorder
DHA	Docosahexaenoic acid (Omega 3 fatty acid)
DR	Diabetes Retinopathy
DR	Doctor
DG	Diabetes Gastropathy
DNA	Deoxyribonucleic acid
DASH Diet	Dietary Approaches to stop Hypertension
DKA	Diabetes Ketoacidosis
DMT1	Diabetes Mellitus Type-1
DMT2	Diabetes Mellitus Type-2
DM	Diabetes Mellitus

EPA	Environmental Protection Agency (USA)
FHS	Follicle Stimulating Hormone
FODMAPS	Fermentable Oligo-di, mono-saccharide and polyols
FSAI	Food Safety Authority of Ireland
FBS	Fasting Blood Sugar
GABA	Gamma Aminobutyric acid
GKI	Glucose Ketone Index
GBM	Glioblastoma Multiforme
GI	Glycemic Index
GL	Glycemic Load
GERD	Gastroesophageal Reflux Disease
HPCSA	Health Profession Council of South Africa
HCA2	Hydroxy – Carboxylic acid receptor 2
HR	Heart Rate
HOMA-IR	Homeostatic Model Assessment of Insulin Resistance
HCTZ	Hydrochlorothiazide
Hs-CRP	Highly sensitive C-reactive protein
HDL-C	High Density Lipoprotein Cholesterol
HbA1c	Hemoglobin A1C
HDL	High Density Lipoprotein
IA2	Islet Antigen 2
IGT	Impaired Glucose Test
IBS	Irritable Bowel Syndrome
IDL	Intermediate Density Lipoprotein
IL-6	Interleukin – 6

IGF – 1	Insulin like Growth Factor-1
IF	Intermittent Fasting
IBD	Inflammatory Bowel Disease
ICU	Intensive Care Unit
IDF	International Diabetes Federation
IR	Insulin Resistance
KD	Ketogenic Diet
LH	Luteinizing Hormone
LSPA	Lifestyle Physical Activity
LGIT	Low Glycemic Index Therapy
LFD	Low Fat Diet
LCD	Low Carbohydrate Diet
LADA	Latent Autoimmune Diabetes of Adulthood
LFTs	Liver Function Tests
LDL-P	Low density Lipoprotein Particles
LDL-C	Low Density Lipoprotein Cholesterol
LDL	Low Density Lipoprotein
LCKD	Low Carb Ketogenic Diet
MODY	Maturity Onset Diabetes of the Young
MCI	Mild Cognitive Impairment
MCRI	Major Combat Related Injury
MRI	Magnetic Resonance Imaging
MAD	Modified Atkins Diet
MTHFR	Methylenetetrahydrofolate Reductase
MTOR	Mammalian target of rapamycin

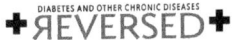
MCT oil	Medium Chain Triglyceride oil
MI	Myocardial Infarction
NLRP3	Inflammasome gene
NCDS	Non Communicable Disease
NBHW	National Board of Health and Welfare
NAFL	Non Alcoholic Fatty Liver
NSAIDS	Non-Steroidal Anti Inflammatory Drugs
NCKD	No Carbohydrate Ketogenic Diet
OGTT	Oral Glucose Tolerance Test
OHA	Oral Hypoglycemic Agents
PET scan	Positron Emission Tomography Scan
PURE Study	Prospective Urban Rural Epidemiology Study
PAH	Pulmonary Arterial Hypertension
PUFS	Polyunsaturated Fats
PCS K9	Enzyme Encoded by PCS K9 Gene
PCOS	Polycystic Ovary Syndrome
QOL	Quality of Life
RA	Rheumatoid Arthritis
RNA	Ribonucleic acid
RCT	Random Control Trial
RBS	Random Blood Sugar
RDA	Recommended Dietary Allowances
SFA	Saturated Fatty Acids
SAD	Standard American Diet
SCS	Seven Countries Study

SD	Standard Diet
SGLT2	Sodium-Glucose Co-Transporter
TBI	Traumatic Brain Injury
TC	Triglyceride
TEI	Total Energy Index
UA	Uric acid
US	United States
USA	United States of America
VLDL	Very Low Density Lipoprotein
VLCD	Very Low Carbohydrate Diet
WBC	White Blood Cell
WFKD	Well Formulated Ketogenic Diet
WHO	World Health Organization

www.ingramcontent.com/pod-product-compliance
Lightning Source LLC
Chambersburg PA
CBHW070526220526
45467CB00003B/877